The Incredible
Secrets of
MUSTARD

Marie Nadine Antol

Foreword by Barry Levenson

D1495479

AVERY PUBLISHING GROUP
Garden City Park • New York

The information contained in this book is based upon the research and the personal experiences of the author. It is not intended as a substitute for consulting with your physician or other health-care provider. The publisher and author are not responsible for any adverse effects or consequences resulting from the use of any of the suggestions or preparations discussed in this book. All matters pertaining to your physical health should be supervised by a health-care professional. It is a sign of wisdom, not cowardice, to seek a second or third opinion.

Cover designer: Doug Brooks
In-house editor: Dara Stewart
Typesetters: Liz Johnson & Gary Rosenberg
Printer: Paragon Press, Honesdale, PA

Avery Publishing Group
120 Old Broadway
Garden City Park, NY 11040
1-800-548-5757
www.averypublishing.com

Cataloging-in-Publication Data

Antol, Marie Nadine
    The incredible secrets of mustard : the quintessential guide to the history, lore,
    varieties, and healthful benefits of mustard / Marie Nadine Antol. — 1st ed.
      p. cm.
    Includes bibliographical references and index.
    ISBN 0-89529-920-8
    1. Cookery (Mustard). 2. Mustard. 3. Mustard (Condiment) I. Title
TX819.M87A58   1999
641.3'384   QBI99-993

Printed in the United States of America

10 9 8 7 6 5 4 3 2 1

Contents

PART TWO   *Mustard Recipes*

This book is dedicated to Joyce Nevin Miller, my friend and neighbor. If we lived in medieval times, Joyce would be the wise woman held in reverence by all in the village. I picture her in a tidy whitewashed cottage, ringed by a weathered cedar fence, with the grounds glorified by a lush and lovely kitchen garden, fragrant with herbs, greens, and vegetables.
In this imaginary medieval village, all who are sick or injured in body or spirit come to consult Goodwife Miller.
None are turned away and all are helped.
This is not so very different from the way it is in the modern-day village where we live.

Joyce not only opened her extensive library to me, she became as fascinated with the subject matter of this book as I am. She provided me with source material for some of the very interesting oddities in this book, and ended up being the best research assistant I have ever had. I am grateful for both her help and her friendship.
This book is all the better for her participation.

Acknowledgments

Thanks go to Barbara Spielberg at the British Consulate in Los Angeles who tracked down the Mustard Museum attached to Colman's Mustard Shop in Norwich, England, after many sources who should have known better told me it didn't exist. Barbara put me in touch with Olive Covell, who provided me with abundant information on the Colman legacy.

Thank you to the American Embassy in Paris, France, for locating Maille's Le Musee Amora in Dijon, and the Maille Mustard Boutique in Paris. Special thanks go to J.D. Bellon in Dijon, who responded to my request for information on the museum with wonderful material and illustrations.

Thanks are due Nancy Noleen of Summers McCann, the firm that handles the Napa Valley Mustard Festival, for conveying to me the very real excitement that mustard brings to the Napa Valley for two months every year.

A huge thank you also goes to Herr G. Weber of Verband der deutschen Senfindustrie e.V., who responded to my query to the Association of the German Mustard Industry with a wealth of information, including facts and figures and mustard preferences throughout Europe.

I am especially grateful to Michael Blaylock, Ph.D., of Phytotech, the pioneering firm that's spearheading the drive to clean up the environment with natural phytoremediation techniques, for documenting the phenomenal power of mustard to leach contaminants from soil and water.

And, finally, applause and thanks to Barry Levenson, curator of the Mount Horeb Mustard Museum and a kindred spirit. The mustard material he shared with me brightened many of my days. Bravo, Barry! Incidentally, I wouldn't have made it through Poupon U and gotten my Doctorate in Mustard without him.

Foreword

I am obsessed with mustard. It has been that way since October of 1986. That's when my beloved Red Sox snatched defeat from the jaws of victory and lost the World Series to the New York Mets. I was devastated.

I could not sleep the night after the fateful seventh game, so I went to an all-night grocery. I walked the aisles, seeking the meaning of life. A new hobby—that's what I needed, something to take my mind off the pain of baseball. As I walked down the condiment aisle, past the ketchups and pickles and hot sauces, I heard a deep resonant voice coming from the mustards: "If you collect us, they will come."

I did, and they have. The Mount Horeb Mustard Museum holds the world's largest collection of mustards (probably more than 3,000 by the time you read this), an impressive array of antique old mustard pots, and lots of mustard memorabilia. Gosh, it really is a museum dedicated to mustard.

Once upon a time, I was a lawyer, arguing criminal cases for the people of Wisconsin in the appellate courts. That was before mustard took over my life. Perhaps my decision to forsake the law in favor of mustard is the best thing I could have ever done for the people of Wisconsin; there's now one less lawyer to worry about.

My most memorable moment as a lawyer came when I argued a case before the United States Supreme Court in 1987. As I left my hotel room to go to court, I noticed a small (1.4-ounce) unopened jar of mustard on a room-service tray in the hallway. The soiled dishes led me (the bright fellow that I was) to conclude that the hotel guests had finished their meal but passed on the mustard.

I consulted my list of mustards (which I always carried with me), and determined that the one before me was one that I did not have. There I was, on my way to the highest court in the land with an ethical dilemma staring me in the face. Is it theft to take an unopened jar of mustard from a discarded room-service tray? I did what every good lawyer would have done. I looked around, saw that no one was watching, and put it in my pocket.

I kept the jar in my left pants pocket. As I argued the case, the mustard gave me great confidence. At the end of my allotted time, Justice Sandra Day O'Connor cleared her throat and asked, "Excuse me, counselor, but is that a jar of mustard in your pocket, or are you just glad to see me?" You can look it up—*Griffin v. Wisconsin*, 483 U.S. 868 (1987). Oh, yes, I won the case.

Books about mustard always excite me. I love to find new techniques for making mustard, new recipes for cooking with mustards, and new ways of using mustards. There are so many different kinds of mustard (we should know!) that the possibilities seem endless. Of course, those are the culinary dimensions of mustard. I am even more thrilled when a mustard book gives something extra—as in history, culture, lore, and adventure.

Nikki Antol has given us lots of extra.

The recipes are fabulous, the suggested uses are imaginative, and the techniques are first-rate. But the extras are the real delight. You may have heard that mustard has been associated with the healing arts for centuries (you may even remember mustard plasters), but you will be delighted as you read what Nikki has discovered about mustard and medicine.

My favorite chapter is the Mustard Miscellany chapter. It could be a whole book by itself (not because it is so long, but because it is so darned fascinating!). Whoever thinks that mustard is blah and one-dimensional will become a true believer in mustard after reading this chapter. Of course, I have always known the virtues of mustard when it comes to uranium detection. Then again, I have emptied my brain of all non-mustard facts, and filled it with only mustard facts (not trivia, thank you). This makes life so much easier.

By the way, did you know that the General Accounting Office

released a report that found that mustard eaters are 44-percent less likely to be audited by the IRS than are mayonnaise eaters (i.e. the "condimentally challenged")?

It is often hard to take mustard seriously, and I suppose I'm not helping things with my often silly approach to it. (Mount Horeb is also the home of America's mustard college—Poupon U!) So-called "gourmet" specialty shops sometimes take a snooty approach to food, which frankly, turns me off. We sell exotic mustards at the museum but try to have fun while we do so. Let's face it: Great mustard is no reason to be uppity, is it?

I must confess that when I started collecting mustards in 1986, I had not even a clue as to how many there were out there or where this journey would lead. I sometimes look back and wonder what would have happened if Bill Buckner had caught that ground ball and the Red Sox had won the World Series. Would I still be a lawyer? Would I have missed the great mustard experience?

It is indeed possible to live without mustard. It's also possible to survive without music, poetry, or art—possible but not much fun. Mustard is an extra that can surprise, delight, and even inspire us. This book is part of that added dimension.

It is said that all true mustard lovers must make a pilgrimage to the Mount Horeb Mustard Museum at least once. (Okay, so I'm the one who said it.) I invite you to come and savor our quirky little establishment. We will swap mustard stories, taste until we drop, tell mustard jokes (there are quite a few!), and in our own way make life's journey a little richer.

This book is now part of that journey—part of the yellow brick road of life.

Barry Levenson, Curator
Mount Horeb Mustard Museum

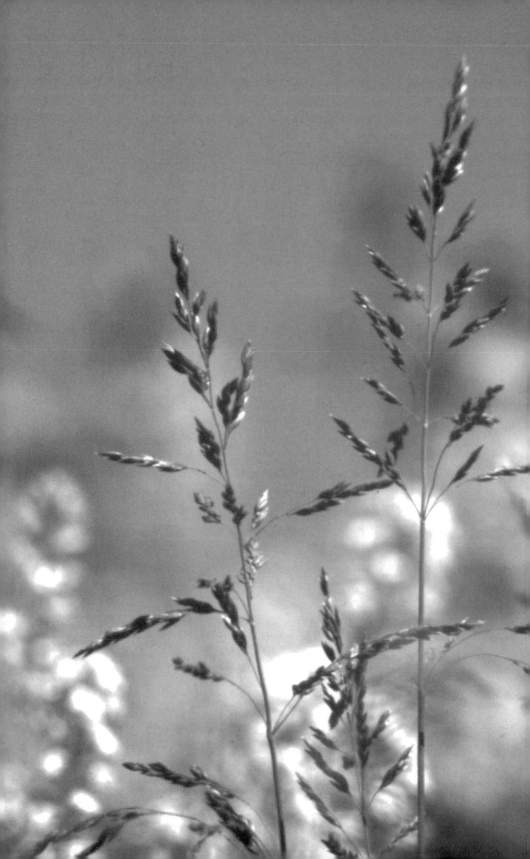

Introduction

The mustard seed and the plant itself have been valued both for their intense flavors and for their healthful properties for centuries. Even in the Bible, there are several references to mustard seeds. Today, most of us think of mustard as only a condiment for hot dogs or pretzels; but there are so many incredible secrets of mustard that most do not know. Here, in *The Incredible Secrets of Mustard*, I present them to you. This book will tell you all there is to know about mustard, including some functions of mustard that I'm sure you never thought of, and provides over fifty tantalizing recipes using mustard seeds and greens and prepared mustards.

This book is separated into two parts. Part One, Mustard Facts, gives you the background of mustard, including its biology, its healthful and medicinal properties, its use throughout history, the varieties of mustard seeds, the types of prepared mustards, and useful applications of mustard.

Part Two, Mustard Recipes, contains useful information for growing your own mustard and recipes for preparing your own mustard creams, as well as recipes that use mustard seeds, greens, and creams.

You are going to have so much fun reading this book! Mustard has such a long, honored, and interesting history. There is so much to learn about it. I hope you enjoy reading about it as much as I enjoyed writing it for you. Enjoy.

Part One
Mustard Facts

As mentioned in the Introduction to this book, mustard has a long and varied history. Part One will tell you all about that history. It provides you with an introduction to the mustard plant, continues with the history of this golden herb, and gives you an in-depth look at how mustard can impact your health. There's also a fascinating chapter that includes some miscellaneous information about mustard, plus a surprising report on how mustard might save this planet from the toxic pollutants that contaminate the soil and water in so many areas. You'll also have a chance to see just how many varieties of prepared mustards are available today. Read on to learn all the secrets of mustard!

1

Meet the Mustard Family

*. . . The kingdom of heaven is like to a grain of mustard
seed, which a man took, and sowed in his field.
Which indeed is the least of all seeds; but when it is grown,
it is the greatest among herbs, and becometh a tree,
so that the birds of the air come and lodge in the
branches thereof.*

—Matthew 13: 31, 32

People have been arguing for centuries over how to categorize mustard. Is it food, medicine, spice, or condiment? Actually, it's all four. Whatever you call it, mustard has been valued for centuries for its warming and stimulating properties, as well as for its pungency and characteristic flavor. Mustard seeds not only help improve digestion, they have recently been discovered to aid in the metabolism of fat. Applied externally, mustard helps relieve chest congestion and joint pain. In later chapters, I'll tell you more about the many ways mustard is used.

The term "mustard" comes from the Middle English word *moustarde*, which was derived from the Old French words *moust* (must) and *ardens*, which means "burning." A moustarde was originally a pungent table relish made from ground mustard seed and must—unfermented juice pressed from grapes or other fruit. So, the forerunner of the popular condiment was a tasty mix of ground mustard seed and fruit juice, and that's not so very different from what we enjoy today.

MUSTARD'S ROOTS

Mustard is prized for its leaves, its seed, and its oil. The leaves of certain varieties of mustard are a spicy addition to a salad, and when the large curly leaves are steamed, they are an exceptionally nutritious green vegetable with a distinctive flavor. In the wild, deer seem to enjoy the flavor of the plant very much.

Either whole or crushed, the seeds have been used by cooks and apothecaries for centuries. Creatures of the wild also enjoy the seeds. For example, the seeds are sought out by ground squirrels and wild birds, including doves, pheasants, woodcock, finches, larks, and nuthatches. Even caged birds appreciate them.

The Mustard Seed

The Bible says mustard is the "least" of all seeds. If you're picturing a mustard seed as the size of a grain of sand, that's not an accurate picture. However, mustard seeds *are* tiny. Perhaps your only use of mustard is of that yellow or brownish stuff you find in jars at your local market. If so, I figure it's up to me to give you a true sense of the size of a mustard seed. In order to do that, I counted the number of the tiniest seeds (black mustard seeds) in a teaspoonful.

First, though, I want you to appreciate the difficulties inherent in my self-imposed task. I measured out a half teaspoonful of seeds and deposited them on a plate. My idea was just to push them into piles of ten with a knife blade, count the piles, and multiply my half teaspoonful of seeds by two to equal a full teaspoonful. Bad idea. The seeds refused to stay in neat little piles. In fact, I couldn't make neat little piles. The seeds rolled everywhere except where I wanted them to roll. Finally, I transferred a few seeds at a time onto another plate with my moistened fingertip, counting as I went. For every ten seeds transferred, I made a line on a piece of scratch paper. Believe me, it stopped being fun long before I was finished. Nonetheless, I am very pleased to be able to tell you that there are 1,654 black mustard seeds in one teaspoon. Now, that's *tiny*.

Mustard seeds have been pressed for their oil for millennia. The Bible itself mentions mustard seeds five times, but other sacred writings also refer to the tiny seed. For example, these words are found in the book of rabbinical writings *The Life and Words of Christ*, compiled by Cunningham Geikie: "There was a stalk of mustard in Sichin from which sprang out three boughs, of which one broke off, and covered the tent of a potter, and produced three cabs [nearly six quarts] of oil." In demonstrating the exceptional fertility of the Promised Land, another rabbinical report cited by Geikie stated, "One man got three hundred-fold increase on the grain of mustard seed he sowed." The theme in all the Biblical references to mustard seed is the same. Out of something minute comes something great.

When the oil is expressed from the seeds, it becomes an indispensable ingredient in some regional dishes, especially those of India, and it's also prized as an ingredient in a powerful massage oil that delivers deep heat. However, the oil is a dangerously caustic irritant. It is so potent, that care must be taken with its use, lest the skin burn and blister. The oil is also used in the manufacture of soap, and in the distant past, mustard oil was sometimes used as fuel in oil lamps.

You may never use a mustard plaster or grow mustard in your garden or grind your own seeds or even enjoy a "mess of mustard greens," but I'm willing to bet that you have a jar or two of mustard in your kitchen. No matter what brand or what flavor of mustard you fancy, it all starts with the seeds. When mustard seeds are finely ground, whether the hulls are left in or sifted out, the resulting powder is the primary ingredient in the familiar condiment. Here's a little centuries-old double-couplet that shows just how much the British, in particular, care about the mustard on the table.

From three things may the Lord preserve us:
From valets much too proud to serve us;
From women smeared with heavy fard, good grief!
From lack of mustard when we eat corned beef.

Of all the flavorings you can name, you might be surprised to learn that only pepper exceeds mustard in popularity around the world.

The Mustard Plant

Wild mustard plants are biennial, meaning that their life cycles last about two years, but only annual strains (those that take a year to grow completely) are cultivated today. Pliny the Elder (A.D. 23–79), the great Roman naturalist who wrote a thirty-seven-volume work called *Historia Naturalis*, noted that mustard grew wild everywhere in Italy without cultivation. He also remarked that the taste of all vegetables was improved by adding a handful of torn mustard greens to the cooking pot. I have found that to be true, and a lot of other people agree with that assessment. Pliny also assured us that mustard is a "virtuous" plant in that it adds nothing toxic to the soil or the system.

The Mustard Tree

The mustard tree cited in the familiar Bible verse that opens this chapter is believed to be from the *Salvadoraceae* family, which contains several evergreen trees and shrubs that have been growing in the Middle East, India, Africa, and China since ancient times. This family includes *S. persica*, which is familiarly called the mustard tree. The mustard tree has bright green leaves that can reach up to two-and-one-half inches in length, and bears small greenish-white bell-shaped flowers, followed by reddish-purple inedible fruits. Although it is not considered a true mustard, the seeds produced by all species of *Salvadoraceae* are rich in volatile mustard oils. While most cultivated mustards are low-growing plants that seldom reach more than three or four feet in height, the mighty mustard tree can attain a height of twenty feet, and its drooping branches make a perfect perch for birds.

THE MUSTARD FAMILY

The plants of the *Brassicaceae* (mustard) family are known as cruciferous plants because of their four-petaled flowers, two short and two long, that resemble a cross. You're undoubtedly familiar with the common cruciferous vegetables broccoli, cabbage, and cauliflower. But you may be surprised to learn that other cruciferous plants include radishes, horseradish, turnips, and cress. Most are very high in sulfur, which adds to the pungency and characteristic odor of these foods.

All seeds derived from the plants of the *Brassicaceae* family contain a rich oil that can be expressed when the seeds are crushed. To the naked eye, the seeds appear perfectly round and smooth. In reality, though, they are finely pitted with pinprick indentations. Mustard seeds contain 30- to 35-percent oil, which makes this member of the *Brassicaceae* family the champion in the oil-yield sweepstakes. The oil carries too much heat to be used medicinally, but it is used in Indian and other cookery. The oil is also used as a lubricant, as an ingredient in soap-making, and as an illuminant—centuries ago, mustard oil was burned in crude oil lamps. When the seeds are ground and the hulls are sifted out, it yields a fine powder or flour. In fact, a package of powdered mustard seeds may be labelled as mustard flour. This very fine powder is used by some commercial manufacturers for making the condiment.

The mustard branch of the cruciferous family tree includes *B. juncea*, variously called brown mustard, Indian mustard, and Chinese (or Oriental) mustard; *B. nigra*, or black mustard; and *B. alba*, also known as *Sinapis alba*, or white mustard. *Sinapis* is the name used by Theophrastus (372–287 B.C.), a Greek philosopher and pupil of Aristotle, in his writings to describe a small genus of mustards cultivated in Asia and Europe. Although the term *Brassica* is preferred today, you'll still see white mustard called *Sinapis alba*, black mustard called *S. nigra*, and brown mustard called *S. juncea* on occasion. In spite of all these slightly different designations, there are just three basic types of mustard: brown, black, and white.

Brown Mustard

Slightly smaller than white mustard seeds and larger than black mustard seeds, brown mustard seeds, *B. juncea*, put forth dark green, upright leaves that measure six to twelve inches long. Small, young leaves are used as green vegetables, much as spinach is used. Brown mustard plants typically top out at around three to four feet. The summer flowers are pale yellow, followed by pods that contain dark golden-yellow seeds. Because *B. juncea* is easily harvested, it's very popular with commercial growers. Brown mustard is grown primarily for its seeds. This is a favorite culinary mustard seed. Although it's recognized as a warming, stimulating herb with mild antibiotic properties, brown mustard is seldom used for medicinal purposes. With only about 70 percent of the pungency of *B. nigra*, brown mustard is considered the mild member of the family.

Black Mustard

The black mustard plant, *B. nigra*, has many branches on each stem, and the leaves are shaped like slender elongated hearts. It produces bright yellow flowers all summer long, followed by small pods. The seeds are about 0.075 inch ($1^1/_2$ millimeters) in size, dark brown, and very pungent. When crushed in water, they give off a sharp, irritating scent. Black mustard plants may reach a height of ten feet, but most grow to around three or four feet. In parts of Great Britain and the United States, the wild plant is considered a troublesome weed. This hot herb stimulates the circulatory and digestive systems, and is a powerful emetic (agent used to induce vomiting) in large doses. Because of its potency, this mustard is preferred for external uses, such as in a mustard plaster. Let the user beware, however. Prolonged contact can cause blistering of the skin.

White Mustard

Herbalists say *Sinapis alba*, white mustard, is a pungent yet gentle mustard seed that stimulates and warms while improving digestion and circulation. It is typically used externally in plasters, poultices, and baths to ease aching joints and for respiratory infections, skin eruptions, and chilblains (a condition in which the hands, feet, and ears itch due to exposure to moist cold). This plant has rough, hairy leaves that grow up to six inches long. The leaves are jagged with irregular cuts. White mustard plants grow upright, but typically attain a height of only two to four feet. Pale yellow flowers, with a surprising vanilla scent, sprout in the summer, followed by pods containing only about three seeds each. The seeds are actually beige (not white) and have a mild flavor. At one-tenth of an inch (2 millimeters) in diameter, though tiny, they are larger than other mustard seeds. White mustard seeds are the primary ingredient in American mustards, and are blended with black mustard seeds to make the typical English mustards. They are not used in French mustards.

THE ESSENCE OF MUSTARD

The characteristic pungency of mustard doesn't develop until cold water is added to the ground seed, and it takes around fifteen minutes for the reaction to occur. If you chew a few mustard seeds, the effect is not the same. The flavor and pungency are still apparent when you crunch the seeds, but in much milder form.

It takes the addition of cold water to mustard powder to initiate a chemical reaction between two constituents of the seed—an enzyme and a substance called a glycoside—which produces the characteristic pungent flavor of mustard seeds. In black and brown mustard, an enzyme called *myrosin* acts on the glycoside *sinigrin* to produce the sulfurous compound *allyl isothiocyanate*. Allyl isothiocyanate is the principal component of the volatile oil expressed from mustard seeds.

With white mustard seeds, the same enzyme acts on a different glycoside, *sinalbin*, to yield sinalbin mustard oil. Unlike black and brown mustard, which carry a whiff of sulfur, the oil of white mustard has very little odor, but it does have a pungent taste. Nonetheless, it is less irritating than the oil obtained from the other members of the family.

No matter what powdered mustard seed is used—brown, black, or white—when hot water or vinegar is used to form the paste, the enzyme is inhibited. The result is a mild, bitter mustard. If you're mixing up powdered Chinese mustard in your kitchen, use very hot water if you want to retain the taste but reduce the pungency and bite. Adding salt also inhibits the enzyme reaction.

Many members of the *Brassica* family have a similar enzyme-and-glycoside reaction in the seeds and, to a lesser degree, in the leaves. Boiling destroys the enzyme. If you're cooking mustard greens and find the taste too intense, cook them twice. Simply discard the original cooking liquid, add fresh water, and boil them again. I'll tell you more about cooking mustard greens in Part Two.

MAKING MUSTARD

Mustard is available in three forms: as seeds, as a dry powder that is freshly mixed with water to obtain the most aroma and flavor, and as a paste or cream blended with vinegar or wine, along with selected spices. Although some mustard seeds are sold whole, most are further processed by grinding. Mustard, whether in seed or powdered form, must be kept dry and cool. Even though the cellular structure remains intact, whole seeds are subject to a slow deterioration of their contents over the passage of time. If you make your own pickles, mustard seed is a necessity. For full flavor, be aware that the whole seed is best used within eighteen months. Mustard powder must not be exposed to the air and must be kept in tightly closed containers. Grinding fractures the cell walls of the seeds, and the seeds will lose volatile constituents. However, if your mustard powder is stored in glass, it will retain most of its properties for up to two years.

Mustard powder and seeds are sold in small containers to the consumer, or in bulk quantities to manufacturers. Bulk buyers include meat packers, fancy sausage specialists, pickle manufacturers, and producers of the familiar condiment in all its many delicious variations.

The basic recipe for "mustard cream" (the condiment we call

Conversational Mustard

Some of the greatest writers of history, including Shakespeare, used mustard to aid in descriptions. For example, in an early reference to mustard's fire and heat, here's a quote from Boswell's *The Life of Samuel Johnson, LLD*: "Johnson's conversation was by much too strong for a person accustomed to obsequiousness and flattery; it was mustard in a young child's mouth." It was in 1791 that James Boswell wrote the celebrated biography of Dr. Johnson that has made both their names immortal.

Between 1880 and 1914 when mustard plasters were in common use, whisperers talking behind the back of a boring young man with a pallid complexion often said he'd be well advised to "put a mustard plaster on his chest." The thought was that a mustard plaster would excite the pale young man, fire him up, and bring a glow to a dull skin and duller personality.

No matter what your age, you're probably acquainted with the phrase "cut the mustard." If someone is able to do something that requires youth and vigor well, he or she is said to be able to "cut the mustard," as in: "He is so good at—whatever—He can really cut the mustard." One source I consulted says this phrase dates back to the early 1900s when the phrases "up to the mustard" (similar to "up to the mark") and "keen as mustard" were in common use. In the 1950s, "mustard" was used to add force when expressing an opinion against something, as in: "This city government is mustard on contamination offenses."

In the 1920s, to be "mustard" was to be very good at something. If the term was applied to a female, as in "Wow! She's really mustard," it signified that the woman was "a hot number," either in appearance or in her bedroom accomplishments (or both). When horses were more common than cars near the end of the nineteenth century, a carriage with a light yellow body was sometimes referred to as a "mustard pot."

Around this same period, lovers who engaged in energetic bedroom acrobatics were said to be really "cutting the mustard." This meaning of the term apparently didn't die out. I came across an isolated quote from an article published in 1978 that said, "It puts its ideological point with admirable concision: pacifists are good in bed; militarists can't cut the mustard."

It's rare to hear "cut the mustard" used in conversation today. If it's used at all, the phrase is most often used negatively, as in: "Too bad. He just can't cut the mustard anymore."

And, finally, who remembers Gene Autry's sidekick, Pat Butram, who added to our delight in all those Saturday afternoon movies? Butram was forever saying "Mustard 'n custard!" in his high-pitched scratchy voice when he was agitated, which was quite often. This expressive phrase is just plain fun to say, especially if you pitch your voice up an octave or two. Try it.

mustard) hasn't changed much over the centuries. You can still buy the powder or the seeds, grind them at home, strain the hulls from the ground seeds, add liquid and spices to the resulting powder, and enjoy the condiment in its purest form. Turmeric is a common addition in commercially prepared mustards. Turmeric is another ancient plant much favored throughout Asia. This herb is pungent and bitter and adds intense yellow color to cream mustards. In some mustards, yellow food coloring takes the place of the turmeric. In milder versions of the condiment, starch or flour may be blended with mustard powder to tone down the sharpness and bite.

Ask any Frenchman, and you'll be told that the mustard capital of the world is Dijon, France. Dijon-style mustards are made from black or brown mustard seeds, which are considered the strongest and most flavorful. After the seeds are ground, white wine is added, along with cloves, cinnamon, and other special herbs and spices. The exact formula for Grey Poupon, arguably the most popular mustard in the universe, is a secret. The recipe is unique and dates back more than 200 years. Nonetheless, in the history of mustard, that makes Grey Poupon a relative newcomer.

MUSTARD TODAY

Mustard greens are a staple in many cultures around the world and are enjoying a rebirth of popularity in the United States. Mustard is often used as a cover crop to hold soil in place, and, when plowed under, serves as a "green manure" that nourishes the soil. It is also cultivated as a nutritious stock feed. When ground, the seeds are used to spice various commercially prepared foods, including cold meats and many forms of sausages. The liquid used for curing pickles usually contains mustard seed, and mustard is also a common ingredient in salad dressings, including dry mixes, and barbeque sauces. And, as you might imagine, in just about every kitchen around the world, you'll find a jar or two of prepared mustard. No household is complete without this familiar golden condiment.

In the next chapter, I'll give you a fast-forward glimpse into the long and honored history of mustard.

— 2 —

Mustard in History

Grumio: What say you to a piece of beef and mustard?
Katharina: A dish I do love to feed upon.
Grumio: Ay, but the mustard is too hot a little.
Katharina: Why then, the beef and let the mustard rest.
Grumio: Nay, then I will not: you shall have the mustard,
  or else you get no beef of Grumio.
Katharina: Then both, or one, or any then thou wilt.
Grumio: Why, then the mustard without the beef.

—The Taming of the Shrew
William Shakespeare (1564–1616)

Back in the sixteenth century when Shakespeare was writing his masterworks with a quill pen, mustard was a common kitchen staple all over the known world, including the American colonies. This hot herb has a very long history. Mustard has been cultivated for millennia, and it's grown throughout most areas of the world. In this chapter, you'll learn all about the history of mustard throughout the world.

ANCIENT CIVILIZATIONS

The *Brassica* family originated in the temperate areas of Asia and the Mediterranean region. Although the name *Sinapis* is of Egyptian origin, the ancient Chinese of 3,000 years ago cultivated several species of mustard in their gardens. According to ancient historical records of China, the hot and spicy seeds were eaten whole with meats and game, not only by the rich at legendary banquets, but by the common people as well, and the greens were eaten fresh or put into soups and stir-fried with common vegetables and just a bit of meat.

One of the earliest references to mustard seed was discovered in cuneiform (a type of ancient writing in which characters are formed by the arrangement of wedge-shaped elements) chiseled on a fragment of a 4,000-year-old clay Sumerian tablet. The characters surrounding the reference to mustard have been lost, so we don't know whether the reference was to mustard as food or medicine; but we do know that the Sumerians used mustard both ways. In case you've forgotten your history, the Sumerians had a thriving culture in Mesopotamia at least as early as the fifth millennium B.C. It has been established that the Sumerians were an agrarian society with a well-developed system of irrigation, and we know that one of the crops they grew was mustard. From remnants of surviving clay tablets, it's apparent that their medicines included mustard, sulfur, opium, licorice, and thyme.

By 1800 B.C., the Babylonians had supplanted the Sumerians in the region. The Babylonians used mustard as part of their many apothecary formulations. The earliest clear recorded use of mustard seeds as food dates back to the Han Dynasty in China, which reigned from 206 B.C. to A.D. 221. According to archeologists, it appears that mustard has served as both food and medicine in China since before recorded history began. India, too, has a long history of using mustard both for its healthful properties and as food. I'll tell you more about its use in Chinese and Ayurvedic medicine in Chapter 3.

Mustard plants are mentioned frequently in early Greek and Roman writings as food, condiment, and medicine. One early anonymous writer declared, "The distressed are quickly cured and the dead resuscitated, thanks to mustard!" Of course, mustard is known to "wake up" the appetite, but there will never be any evidence that it can awaken the dead. Apicus, the Roman author of the cookbook *De Re Coquinaria*, gave recipes for preparing "sinapi confecta," which resembles the condiment we enjoy today, as well as instructions for preparing dishes that included "sinapi confecta" among the ingredients. For example, here's Apicus' sauce for boar: "Grind and mix mustard, pepper, caraway, lovage, grilled coriander seeds, dill, celery, thyme, oregano, onion, honey, vinegar, fish stock and oil. Baste the spitted boar regularly." Surprisingly, there was no mention of putting an apple in the boar's mouth!

The ancient Greeks held the mustard seed and its medicinal properties in such high esteem that they attributed the discovery of mustard to Asclepius, the legendary Greek god of medicine. Mustard seed was also prescribed medicinally by Hippocrates (460–370 B.C.), who is considered to be the father of medicine. Aristotle (384–322 B.C.) is said to have insisted that game, such as goose, duck, thrush, and quail, be roasted with mustard to heighten its flavor before he would permit such dishes to be served at his table. Theoprastus (372–287 B.C.), who succeeded Aristotle as head of the school he founded, is known to have cultivated several varieties of mustard in his garden, perhaps because he often had Aristotle as a guest for dinner. In the first century A.D., Pedanius Dioscorides, a famous Greek physician of the day, wrote extensively on substances used in medicine, with mustard often playing a starring role in his writings. Dioscorides' *De materia medica* eventually totaled five volumes with approximately 1,000 remedies, and it remained the leading pharmacological text for sixteen centuries. The original Greek manuscript was copied by scribes into at least seven other languages. The last publication of *De materia medica* was the English translation, which came out in 1934.

In recent years, Egyptologists have discovered mustard seeds packed in elaborate jars in tombs, an indication that they were used as ritual offerings to the gods in ancient times. We also know that the ancient Egyptians, as well as the Greeks and Romans, ate the seeds whole. The usual custom was to take a bite of meat, drop a few seeds into the mouth, and chew. I tried sprinkling whole mustard seeds on a turkey sandwich and found each bite quite good. Some scholars have suggested that part of the popularity of pungent mustard might be attributed to its ability to mask the taste of spoiled food.

Over a thousand years ago, Swedish vikings began a tradition that survives to this day. The thin mustard sauce used to glaze *julskinka* (a Christmas ham) began as a type of sacrifice to Frey, the goddess of love. The mustard glaze was used on wild game back then. Today, the glaze dresses holiday hams. Herring dressed with mustard sauce (*sennepssild*) is a very old Danish delicacy that is still enjoyed today. The mustard sauce (*sennepssauce*) Danes have used for centuries as a dressing for meat and fish consists of meat or fish stock boiled with dry mustard, vinegar, sugar, and paprika. I'm sure you've recognized the similarity between the Danish word *senneps* and the word for mustard—*sinapis*—which was coined by the Egyptians, and which we still use today.

EUROPE

The cultural Renaissance that began in Italy in the fourteenth century and spread throughout Europe saw the birth of "criers," those merchants who trundled their wares on wheelbarrows throughout the streets, door to door. By the 1600s, every city in Europe, including those of the British Isles, had wheelbarrow or pushcart merchants in the streets. These tradesmen hawked their goods to humble housewives, as well as the gentry. There were "criers" who, along with bread and milk, meat and fish, and fruit and vegetables, specialized in what were called "hellish" spices and sauces, which, of course, included mustard. (See Figure 2.1 below.)

It wasn't long before mustard-makers began competing with one another for the privilege of becoming a supplier to one of the crowned heads of empires. It was a supreme honor to make mustard for the imperial court. During this period 1,001 new recipes for mustard were created, with each mustard-maker hoping his mustard would catch the favor of his sovereign. It was a race to see who would receive a license to supply the court. Finding favor with the king was as good as money in the bank. Once a mustard-maker was able to label his product "by appointment to his majesty," sales to the surrounding gentry skyrocketed.

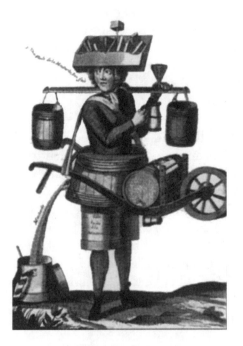

Figure 2.1.
A peddler of "hellish" sauces, circa 1700.
Courtesy of Le Musée Amora, Dijon, France.

Italy

In fourteenth-century Italy, *mostarda di frutta* was served with meat and game. This condiment was prepared by preserving large chunks of assorted fruits in a thin, sweet, very fiery mustard syrup. From all accounts, mostarda di frutta was a particular favorite of the Dukes of Milan. It's still made much the same way today, and you can still find mostarda di frutta in gourmet shops and specialty catalogs.

France

In Paris, mustard-makers appeared on the royal registers for the first time in 1292. Businesses had to follow certain guidelines in the making of their products to appear on the royal registers. Those registered companies were the most sought after. A royal edict dating back to 1351 cites that mustard makers and sellers were among those select merchants who were permitted to possess weights to weigh their wares for sale. In medieval times, the French pounded mustard seeds in a mortar and pestle, sometimes straining out the hulls and sometimes not. The resulting powder, coarse or fine, was then mixed with honey and vinegar or fruit juice.

Whatever method was used, the honor of making the first crock of "mustard cream" probably belongs to France. It's been written that guests at a gala given by the Duke of Burgundy in 1336 consumed 70 gallons of prepared mustard in one sitting! I bet you won't be at all surprised when I remind you that Dijon, home of master mustard-makers for centuries, is the historic capital of Burgundy.

Burgundy, land of vineyards and fine wine, was uniquely situated to provide its *moutarde*-makers with the necessary wine or vinegar needed to produce particularly fine varieties of the condiment. (See Figure 2.2 on page 20.) The area was also populated with charcoal makers, who themselves contributed to mustard-making in a roundabout way. The charcoal was produced in vast glades. Its production added a lot of potassium to the soil, which was highly favorable to the growth of mustard. Plants grown in this rich soil flourished. Due to all this industry in the region, many residents of Burgundy were wealthy, and just about all the townspeople were comfortably well off. They could afford to eat meat and mustard at every meal. Thus, the mustard-makers had heavy consumers. All the components necessary for a superb symbiotic relationship were

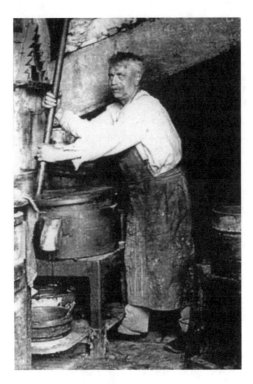

Figure 2.2.
Fabricating moutarde
in 1850.
Courtesy of Le Musée Amora,
Dijon, France.

in place, from plants to seeds to ingredients to consumers. It's no wonder that Dijon is still known for its mustard today.

In the fourteenth century, the canon of the cathedral of Lille, France, Jehan Millot, compiled a listing of old proverbs. He recorded this gem in his collection: "There is but one town with the name Dijon. There is no mustard but the one from Dijon." By the middle of the seventeenth century, the mustard-makers of Dijon, France, had organized themselves into a guild to protect the purity and to insure the quality of the finished product. Mustard was such serious business in France that members of the mustard guild were forbidden to have more than one shop. That way, if a less-than-perfect batch of mustard reached the marketplace, its origin was easy to track. Undoubtedly, if that ever happened, the offender's reputation would have been ruined, as in: "You'll never make mustard in this town again! Get out!" France is still serious about mustard.

Dijon mustard is arguably the most popular mustard in the United States these days. When you consider that the master mustard-makers of Dijon, France, have been renowned since the thirteenth century, perhaps that's not surprising. An anonymous historian wrote, "The 18th century consecrated Dijon as the universal mustard capital." That tradition continues today. The French are so fond of mustard that they call it the "condiment of kings," and have even passed strict laws governing which mustard creams could aspire to the proud Dijon name. Dijon mustards must adhere to "appellation controllee" standards, which regulate allowable ingredients in and manufacturing methods of products. The controls are as strict for mustard as they are for fine French wines.

Thanks in part to their clever "Pardon me, do you have any Grey-Poupon?" advertising, the most famous of the great Dijon mustard firms today is Grey-Poupon, which was founded in 1777. The company was started when Monsieur Grey developed a unique recipe for a strong mustard made with fine white wine; however, he very much wanted to develop a wider market. Unfortunately, to do it right, he needed more francs than he had, so he invited Monsieur Poupon to join him. It was Grey who made the mustard, and Poupon who supplied the financial backing for the venture. This was truly a marriage made in mustard-heaven. Monsieurs Grey and Poupon went on to revolutionize mustard-making by introducing the first automatic mustard-making machine. The rest, as they say, is history.

If you don't recognize the name, you don't know mustard. Incidentally, if you want to visit what the Grey-Poupon people like to think of as the "mecca of mustard lovers," drop in on Grey-Poupon at 32 Rue de la Liberté, in the heart of Dijon, France.

England

Some sources believe that Roman garrisons brought mustard to England, eating it with their camp meals and sowing the seeds on their marches. Other historians maintain that mustard seed came to the British Isles in the droppings of migratory birds (not in the droppings of Roman centurions), although both versions probably have truth to them. However it happened, the early Britons took mustard to their hearts. They used the greens as potherbs, and ate the seeds, whole or ground and mixed with liquid and "fixings," and slathered the resulting mustard cream over their meats.

"Instant" mustard cream was an early development. British housewives ground mustard seeds coarsely, added some flour and a little cinnamon, moistened the powder, and rolled it into balls. After drying, the mustard balls were easy to store. When the lady of the house wanted to serve mustard cream, the balls were broken up and mixed with vinegar or wine, adding to the flavor.

Tewkesbury, a market town in Gloucestershire, England, was famous for its mustard balls. Tewkesbury mustard balls were so well known that they were immortalized by Shakespeare. In *King Henry the Fourth*, Shakespeare wrote, "He a good wit? Hang him, baboon! His wit's as thick as Tewkesbury mustard." In 1657, an English herbalist named Coles wrote: "In Glostershire about Teuxbury they grind Mustard seed and make it up into balls which are brought to London and other remote places as being the best that the world affords." In his *Acetaria*, written in 1699, John Evelyn recommended the "best Tewkesbury or the soundest and weightiest Yorkshire seeds" for mustard-making. The popularity of this special mustard has endured. You can still buy it today.

Evelyn was also interested enough in all things pertaining to mustard that he took pains to record the fact that the Italians of his day preferred the ground seeds of black mustard blended with orange and lemon peel, a version of which—the mostarda di frutta mentioned earlier—is still found in specialty shops.

For several centuries after Shakespeare hung up his quill, mustard was made up into balls with spices, honey, or vinegar added to keep until they were needed. At the close of the eighteenth century, one Mrs. Clements, a housewife of Durham, England, became famous for her very special, very finely ground mustard powder. Mrs. Clements ground her mustard seeds in a hand mill, then sifted the flour to remove the hulls, and sold the fine powder for a fine profit. Amazingly, no one caught on. She kept her "secret process"—which consisted of merely sifting out the hulls—a deep, dark secret for many years. For a very long time, Mrs. Clements' mustard flour was sold under the name of "Durham Mustard."

J. and J. Colman, established in 1814, was already one of Britain's premiere mustard manufacturers when the company joined forces with Reckitt & Sons, a maker of starch and flour, which was founded in 1840. These two British firms united in 1913. Although the company has diversified, it continues to produce Colman's mustard, which remains a very popular brand of English mustard today. In 1926, Reckitt & Colman bought the R.T. French Company, which had been established in 1880 as a spice company. French's yellow mustard remains one of the most familiar of all basic mustards in the supermarket today.

When burgeoning trade brought exotic spices to Britain and Europe in the sixteenth century, the pervasive use of mustard dropped off. Nonetheless, mustard never lost its popularity, and it's still a staple in British households today.

AMERICA

Although there's no evidence that colonists traveling to the New World on the Mayflower carried mustard seeds, we do know that later travelers brought seeds and cultivated the plants. It's been reported that early Spanish priests sowed mustard seeds to mark their trails from one mission to another along the coast of California.

Undoubtedly, both the spicy taste of the greens and the pungency of the seeds of this hot herb were very welcome in the New World, but it was also considered a premier medicinal. Mustard plasters were used to treat coughs and colds and to break up catarrh, an inflammation of the respiratory tract that produces heavy phlegm. Ague, a feverish condition characterized by severe chills that caused shivering and aching bones, also yielded to mustard's medicinal properties.

And finally, just in case you were wondering, mustard first met the hot dog at the 1904 St. Louis World's Fair when the R.T. French Company introduced its popular version of cream mustard. Now, everyone knows that hot dogs and mustard just naturally go together. Dave Barry, a contemporary American Pulitzer-Prize-winning humorist whose syndicated column is widely applauded, once wrote a satirical piece entitled, "Test Students on Subjects That Matter the Most." I love his sense of the ridiculous.

Barry suggests that students should be tested on "five basic disciplines: English, mathematics, science, history, and condiments." On Barry's proposed test, the condiments section includes this question: "What goes on a hot dog?" Answer: "Mustard." In the science section, Barry asks, "What is the smallest unit of matter?" Answer: "The amount of mustard they put in those condiment packets that you have to open with your teeth." In Barry's test, history and mathematics are combined. The question is: "If Abraham Lincoln is writing the Declaration of Independence at 20 words per minute on a train traveling west from San Francisco, and at exactly the same time, Teddy Roosevelt is forming the National League of Nations on a train traveling east from Boston, what should they put on their hot dogs?" Answer: "Mustard. And they had better do it quickly before their trains hit the ocean." The English section of Barry's test even has a provision for extra credit, to wit: "Make repeated references to mustard."

Not surprisingly, this book makes "repeated references to mustard." I wonder if Dave Barry would deem my efforts worthy of extra credit. Well, I love Dave Barry's writing; it can really cut the mustard.

MUSTARD POTS

A fourteenth-century document makes mention of a mustard pot, although special containers set aside just for mustard were probably in use before then. Because the wheelbarrow vendors sold their mustard by the ladleful, the housewife (or the kitchen maid) making the purchase was required to present a container to hold the mustard cream as it was ladled out, even if it was just a cracked teacup. The mustard pot was an indispensable item in every household. Whether made of wood, clay, glass, pewter, or silver, mustard pots have graced the table in countless homes for well over 500 years and counting.

By the end of the 1700s, when mustard had evolved into a commodity for sale, mustard pots were small earthenware containers made of fine, reddish clay, glazed with a hard white finish. These little pots were not decorated, but the name and address of the manufacturer were inscribed on them with a goose quill. In Dijon, France, the favorite mustard pot was tall with a narrow neck, a curved rim, and a cork stopper. (See Figure 2.3 below.) Because the demand for Dijon mustard was so great, identifying the mustard-maker with a

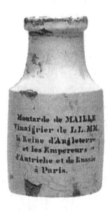

Figure 2.3.
Glazed mustard pot
hand-inscribed with
the maker's name.
Courtesy of Le Musée
Amora, Dijon, France.

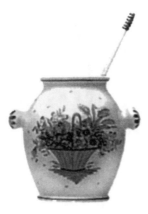

Figure 2.4.
Glazed mustard pot decorated with a stencil.
Courtesy of Le Musée Amora, Dijon, France.

handwritten message was no longer practical. It was much faster to use a stencil, and the decorative motifs that had come into fashion were done with a print roller. (See Figure 2.4 above.)

By the nineteenth century, faience and delft pots filled with mustard had found their way into the marketplace. Faience, which originally was a designation given to pottery produced in Faenza, Italy, since the fourteenth century, is particularly fine earthenware or pottery decorated with colorful glazes. Delft evolved in the sixteenth century in Delft, Netherlands. It was pottery with an opaque glaze, decorated, usually with blue and white, in Oriental style. Before long, many manufacturers had begun producing faience, and soon companies all over Europe were competing with one another to produce fancy mustard pots, which are considered highly collectable today. The advent of indelible transfers made it possible to include a registered trademark, address, specialty, and any awards received by the mustard-maker in competitions and fairs. Mustard-makers who received awards capitalized on their expertise and promoted themselves ferociously on their jars.

The earliest surviving metal examples of mustard pots, typically fashioned with domed lids and pedestal bases, date from the seventeenth century. The hinged lids were opened by depressing a lever on the handles with the thumb. The lids had a small opening cut in the opposite side that held a small spoon for dipping out an individual serving. The earliest surviving metal mustard spoons date from the middle of the eighteenth century. Many of the finest pots were adorned with elaborate decorations, which might include etching and gold inlays.

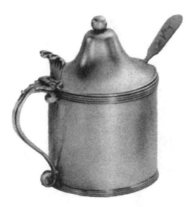

Figure 2.5.
Cobalt-glass lined sliver
mustard pot and spoon.
English, 1790.

Because mustard is so strongly acidic, it cannot be kept in un-protected metal. The pots were lined with pottery or glass, and the spoons had to be removed, washed, and dried after the meal was finished. (See Figure 2.5 above.) For centuries, no table was complete without a mustard pot. The wealthy had a selection of mustard pots, usually made of fine silver and lined with cobalt glass, but no manor house was considered well outfitted unless it also had some not-so-fine pots for the staff. While aristocrats fancied silver mustard pots, the gentry had pewter, and the peasants made do with pottery.

Today, we bring our mustard home from the market in glass jars, or plastic squeeze bottles. Nineteenth-century Europeans would be amazed.

In the next chapter, I'll tell you why the use of mustard as medicine has survived since ancient times. This hot herb has some amazing properties, as you will see.

3

Mustard and Your Health

" . . . and the fruit thereof shall be for meat,
and the leaf thereof for medicine."

—Ezekiel 47:12

Many plants familiar to us today were used medicinally in Biblical times. Mustard was used extensively in the ancient world, both internally and externally. For example, records survive showing that in Biblical times, mustard seeds were used for their laxative properties and to treat indigestion. These tiny seeds were prized for their ability to stimulate the intestinal tract. The treatment included drinking a lot of water.

Ancient healers also prescribed mustard poultices to treat complaints of the lungs, liver, and kidneys, as well as to relieve aches and pains. In the Middle Ages, mustard was used against asthma, coughs, and chest congestion. Small amounts of the ground seeds mixed with water were recommended to relieve acid indigestion and to treat chronic constipation. Ancient healers also discovered that when a great quantity of ground seed was ingested with water, it caused vomiting, making it a useful emetic to combat poisoning. Mustard oil, expressed from the hulls of seeds, was said to be a cure for baldness when rubbed into the scalp.

There is some question in the minds of historians as to whether India or China was the first to develop a viable system of medicine using natural botanicals; however, we do know that these ancient medical protocols developed independently of each other. Both the ancient art of Chinese medicine and the Ayurvedic traditions of India have survived for millennia, and healers of both of these ancient civilizations knew the value of mustard.

TRADITIONAL CHINESE MEDICINE

The Chinese system of medicine is centuries old. According to legend, it began with Fu Hsi, the first of China's emperors, around 2953 B.C. The Yellow Emperor Huang Ti, who died in 2598 B.C., was the author of a great work called the *Nei Ching*. Most ancient Chinese medical literature is founded on this work, and it is still considered authoritative today. The basic tenet of Chinese medicine is the theory of yin and yang. Yang, the male principle, is active and light; yin, the female principle, is passive and dark. The Chinese believe that health, character, and success are determined by the balance of the yin and yang. The great aim of Chinese medicine is to control the proportions of yin and yang within the body.

In China, food *is* medicine. Centuries after the *Nei Ching* was written, Hippocrates said, "Let your food be your medicine; let your medicine be your food," but the Chinese were the first to put this belief into practice. In China, not only does food provide the nutrients the body requires for good health, but Chinese healers use certain foods both to prevent and to treat illnesses. Practitioners of Traditional Chinese Medicine believe that "regulating foods" control the internal environment and act to reduce "immune excess," defined as the body's overreaction to an attack by foreign agents.

Mustard is considered one of the supreme regulating foods. It increases the circulation of energy, warms the internal region of the body, disperses colds, removes phlegm, treats coughs and sore throats, and is good for easing abdominal pain. The ancient Chinese also used mustard to induce vomiting.

Mustard is considered especially valuable for expelling sputum from the lungs. The amount, color, and contents of sputum are important in the diagnosis of many illnesses. Practitioners of Traditional Chinese Medicine teach that the presence of sputum in the body is due to conditions of the internal environment. The presence of sputum is believed responsible for many diseases, including localized swellings that are neither itchy nor painful; lumps in the breast; mucous discharge; hard spots in the abdomen; gastric distress; intestinal obstructions with fluid retention; goiter; swollen lymph nodes; and breast, liver, and stomach cancer. The ancient strategy for eliminating sputum in the body centers on eating the right foods.

Foods that are used to eliminate sputum are called expectorant foods. They include white or brown mustard seeds and the leaves of brown mustard.

Practitioners of Traditional Chinese Medicine believe that poor energy circulation can affect various vital organs and can cause pain. Symptoms arising from poor energy circulation are collectively called "energy congestion," and may give rise to such symptoms as chest pain and congestion, abdominal pain and swelling, hernias, cystitis, hepatitis, menopausal melancholia (major depression), gastrointestinal disorders, peptic ulcers, ringing in the ears, urination difficulties, and uterine bleeding.

Mustard seeds and the leaf of brown mustard are on the list of foods that promote energy circulation in Chinese medicine. China boasts many different varieties of brown mustard. In China today, brown mustard seed is still used to treat colds, stomach problems, abscesses, rheumatism, lower-back pain, and ulcers. The leaves are used to treat bladder inflammation.

Another way that Chinese healers use food as medicine is in the famed Chinese medicinal porridges, or *congees*. Congee is a thin porridge or gruel composed primarily of herbs, vegetables, and rice, although other grains may also be used. Because they are light and easy to digest, and do not overburden the stomach and intestines, they are particularly suitable for invalids and convalescents. The first written record of these very special medicinal porridges dates back to the Han Dynasty (206–220 B.C.). Throughout the history of Chinese medicine, congees have been the backbone of many treatments.

In the third century A.D., during the reign of the Eastern Jin Dynasty, Ge Hong, a Taoist saint and doctor, said, "To prolong life, it is essential to keep the stomach and intestines clear." In the seventh century A.D., Sun Si-Miao, a famed doctor of the Tang Dynasty, said that the superior doctor should first change his patient's diet and lifestyle before resorting to treatment. He claimed that "Old people who eat congee all day keep their body strong and fortified and enjoy great longevity." Dr. Sun called congee "a prescription worth a thousand pieces of gold." On page 43, you'll find a recipe for congee that uses mustard greens. You may keep your thousand pieces of gold. No charge.

AYURVEDIC MEDICINE

Ayurvedic medicine has been practiced in India for over 5,000 years. It is a highly personalized system of medicine that uses natural therapies to keep the mind, the body, and the spirit healthy and to restore the natural harmony of the individual. The earliest concepts of Indian medicine are set out in sacred writings called the Vedas, especially in the passages of the Atharvaveda, which may date back as far as 3,500 years. According to surviving records, the system of medicine called Ayurveda, which means "science of life," was received from the gods by a personage named Dhanvantari, who was himself deified as the god of medicine. The Vedas are rich in treatments for fever; cough; consumption (now referred to as pulmonary tuberculosis); diarrhea; dropsy (now referred to as edema); abscesses; seizures; tumors; and skin diseases, including leprosy. The herbs recommended for these conditions are numerous.

Those who practice Ayurvedic medicine believe that the body contains three elementary substances—spirit (air), phlegm (sputum), and bile. Ancient Vedic healers taught that the health of the body is dependent on the normal balance of the three divine universal forces enumerated above. Indian therapeutic treatment was based first on diet, which was adjusted before any medicinal intervention was attempted. The materia medica (substances used in the preparation of drugs) of the ancients were extensive and consisted mainly of vegetable drugs, all of which were drawn from indigenous plants. Healers collected and prepared their own remedies.

In this system of medicine, the "Actions of the Tastes" plays a basic role. Foods that are pungent, such as mustard, are considered stimulating, carminative (gas expelling), and diaphoretic (sweat inducing). Pungent foods are credited with regulating the metabolism, improving all organic functions, and promoting good digestion. Ancient Indian healers believed that the blending of specific tastes resulted in specific actions. For example, the Ayurveda teaches that pungent (mustard) and bitter (aloe) tastes combine well to promote drying and cleansing. Pungent combined with sour (yogurt) and salty (seaweed) tastes help stimulate digestion. Pungent aids the digestion of sweet (sugar), while sweet helps alleviate the burning sensation caused by pungent tastes.

Conditions caused by byproducts of inefficient digestion, which causes an accumulation of undigested food and waste matter, are called "Ama" conditions. Ama conditions are evidenced by a coated tongue, bad breath, foul body odor, upset stomach, distended abdomen, and feelings of heaviness and dullness. In Sanskrit, *sa* means "with." Thus, a person with an Ama condition was said to be Sama, or with Ama. The Ayurveda teaches that Sama therapies are indicated until these conditions clear. Ancient writings warn that during the process of detoxification, toxins are released, which may cause headaches or other side effects.

When selecting herbs for the detoxification process, sweet, salty, and sour tastes should be avoided because they increase Ama and feed toxins. However, pungent and bitter tastes are effective against Sama. Bitter reduces it. Pungent destroys it. The main Ayurvedic method of treating Sama is the use of herbs that increase digestive fire, thus "burning" it. Herbs that stimulate and that are fiery in nature are used. Best are the hot spices, such as mustard, cayenne, black pepper, dry ginger, long pepper, and asafoetida, which is a soft gummy resin obtained from the roots of plants of the genus *Ferula*. Many Asian species of this family yield strongly scented medicinal resins.

Vedic teachings recommend avoiding mucus-forming foods during any form of respiratory distress, but say hot spices (mustard, cayenne, ginger, and pepper) can be used freely. Ayurveda teaches that the formation of mucus is inhibited by pungent tastes. For arthritis and circulatory disorders, the hot herbs are used in pastes or plasters, and sugar, dairy, and fatty foods are forbidden. These ancient healers recommended applying mustard, camphor, or cinnamon oil to the chest to break up congestion. According to the tradition, the chanting of *Om* will increase the effectiveness of the remedy.

Ayurvedic medicine is now practiced all over the world. These teachings of India became the basis of the healing traditions of many Buddhist lands, and it is believed that Ayurvedic medicine even influenced early Roman and Greek physicians.

ANCIENT GREEK MEDICINE

Hippocrates (460–370 B.C.), known as the Father of Medicine

because of his scientific approach to healing, prescribed mustard seed for use internally and as a poultice. Accounts survive showing that he treated many lung conditions, including all types of respiratory distress, with a mustard plaster made with vinegar instead of water. For millennia, Greek physicians routinely prescribed mustard plasters to break up lung congestion. He also administered mustard frequently in disorders of the digestive organs. Hippocrates' writings appeared in translation all over the known world, and are still highly regarded today.

In the first century A.D., perhaps with an assist from the historical Hippocrates, the Greek physician and pharmacologist Pedanius Dioscorides wrote: "Mustard is good in general for any pain of long continuance when we would draw out anything from deep within to the outside of the body." The text included instructions for making and applying a mustard plaster. Dioscorides is the author of *De materia medica*, which was a leading pharmacological text for sixteen centuries. Dioscorides was an acknowledged authority on botanical medicine.

Mustard seed was also once considered an antidote for various deadly substances, including poisonous mushrooms and hemlock, probably because it can induce vomiting. You may remember that Socrates (469–399 B.C.) died of hemlock poisoning. Socrates is credited with being one of the wisest men of his time, but his ideas threatened certain powerful Athenians. After a trumped-up trial, which resulted in a death sentence, he is reported to have quaffed a cup of poison hemlock "with noble calm and courage." Because Socrates was an honorable man, we have to assume that he would have refused to take mustard as an antidote, had it been offered.

EUROPEAN MEDICINE

The British Pharmacopoeia once listed a Compound Liniment of Mustard, which was described as a very useful application for chronic rheumatism, congestion, colic, and chilblain. Chilblain is an inflammation of the hands and feet caused by exposure to cold and moisture. The Compound Liniment of Mustard was composed of oil of mustard dissolved in spirit of camphor. Camphor itself is rather powerful. This liniment must have generated a terrific amount of heat.

As early as the fifth century A.D., the Anglo-Saxons of the British Isles used mustard plasters for congestion and all respiratory distress. Throughout the Middle Ages and beyond, respected European healers of the day prescribed mustard plasters to relieve aches and pains, including those of the joints. A mustard poultice remained a favorite remedy for arthritis for centuries.

Throughout Europe and the Balkan States and as far east as Russia, white mustard seeds were once a fashionable remedy as a laxative, especially for older people. It was recommended that one chew one-half ounce of whole white mustard seeds. Unfortunately, instead of chewing the seeds, many people swallowed them whole. When it was suspected that taking the seeds whole caused inflammation of the stomach and intestinal tract, this remedy fell into disfavor. However, mustard did relieve chronic constipation, so healers prescribed mustard powder dissolved in water instead of the whole seeds.

Many herbalists have written about the wonders of mustard. At one time or another in its long history, mustard has been used as a remedy for accidental poisonings and snakebite, with the following caveat: "if it be taken in time."

A renowned British herbalist of the eighteenth century named Parkinson wrote, "Mustard is of good use, being fresh, for Epilepticke persons . . . if it be applyed hot inwardly and outwardly." Old herbal texts state that chewing mustard seeds will relieve a toothache, and one old herbal book stated that an infusion (tea) of the seeds will relieve chronic bronchitis and rheumatism. This same source said, "Mustard is of service in the alleviation of neuralgia and other pains and spasms . . . and a gargle of Mustard Seed Tea will relieve and relax a sore throat."

In 1699, British herbalist John Evelyn wrote in his *Acetaria,* "Mustard is of incomparable effect to quicken and revive the spirits . . . besides being an approved antiscorbutic," which is a reference to mustard's ability to conquer scurvy. Today we know that this nutritious plant provides a lot of vitamin C, which is well established as both a preventer of and a cure for scurvy.

MUSTARD AND YOUR HEALTH TODAY

Most knowledgeable health authorities recommend that we eat five to six servings of green leafy vegetables every day. Green leaves that are good for us include mustard greens, of course, as well as spinach, kale, Swiss chard, Chinese cabbage, and the greens of dandelions, beets, collards, and turnips. Mustard greens compare favorably with all the other green leafy vegetables in nutrient content, and they're better tasting than some of those others.

For example, in one pound of mustard greens, you'll get a healthy 581 milligrams of calcium. One of the nicest things I can tell you about enjoying a heaping helping of mustard greens is that this plant doesn't contain large amounts of oxalic acid, and that's what makes it a richly delicious source of calcium. Oxalic acid interferes with the body's absorption of calcium. Spinach, Swiss chard, and beet greens, as delicious as they are, cannot be considered good sources of calcium because these greens are loaded with oxalic acid.

Eat heartily. One pound of mustard greens contains only 98 calories and just one tiny gram of fat. A half-cup serving contains 1,484 international units of vitamin A, 52.5 micrograms of folic acid, 19.6 milligrams of vitamin C, and 99.12 milligrams of potassium. If you eat the whole pound, you'll take in 17.8 grams of complex carbohydrates, 159 milligrams of phosphorus, 9.6 milligrams of iron, 30 milligrams of thiamine (vitamin B_1), 0.69 milligrams of riboflavin (vitamin B_2), and 2.8 milligrams of niacin (vitamin B_3), plus traces of sulfur, iron, cobalt, manganese, and iodine, and a whopping 308 milligrams of vitamin C (ascorbic acid).

Learn from the knowledge of the ancients. Taken internally, hot and pungent herbs, such as mustard, act as expectorants. They help to thin the lung's secretions so they can be coughed up and expelled. When mustard hits the stomach, the theory is that the nerves send a signal to the vagus nerve in the brain, which in turn transmits a message to the lungs, which causes the bronchial glands to release additional fluid. The increased fluid production not only thins the mucus, but actually inhibits the mucus-producing glands so that mucus flows more easily and is easier to cough up and expel. Mustard helps cleanse the entire respiratory tract by breaking up nasal and lung congestion and by clearing the sinuses. The extra fluid production stimulated by mustard also helps flush away irritants. The ancients got it right. If you have a cold, sinus problems, lung congestion, asthma, or bronchitis, try eating hot, pungent foods.

Internally, mustard causes a slight inflammation that causes the blood vessels to dilate, thus increasing blood flow in the area. This slight irritation of the tissues occurs in the mouth, esophagus, and stomach and causes an increase in the production of digestive juices, which aids digestion. When the constituents of mustard are absorbed into the bloodstream, they stimulate blood flow in all tissues, which causes the familiar sensation of flushing and perspiration that can occur after eating a hot, spicy meal. These effects are what make mustard a warming food.

In spite of its many wonderful properties, when taken in large quantities, it's been shown that mustard has the potential to slow down thyroid function. For that reason, people with hypothyroidism (sluggish thyroid) should avoid excessive use of this condiment. That doesn't mean you can't have mustard on your sandwich or enjoy its flavor in cookery, it just means that you shouldn't take a spoonful every day.

Today, science has determined that mustard plasters used externally are effective in easing inflammations that occur below the surface of the skin. Mustard is a rubefacient herb that works as a counterirritant. The term "rubefacient" comes from the Latin *rubeus*, or red, and *facient*, also Latin, meaning "that which causes." So, a rubefacient substance is something that brings blood to the surface and causes the skin to redden. This means that when applied externally, mustard causes the blood vessels to dilate, and brings blood rushing to the area, causing the skin to redden. The increased blood supply helps carry away the toxins that caused the original inflammation. While warming the area, mustard also acts to relieve pain, ease sore muscles, and help loosen up stiff joints.

Although many consider mustard nothing more than a folk remedy, it's still listed in some medical dictionaries. For example, *Taber's Cyclopedic Medical Dictionary* describes mustard seed thus: "Yellow powder of mustard seed is used as a counterirritant [an agent that causes irritation to counter already present inflammation], rubefacient, emetic, stimulant, and condiment."

There are even some drugs in use today that are related to mustard. For example, the *Physicians' Desk Reference* (more familiarly known as the *PDR*) lists Mustargen as a "nitrogen analog of sulfur mustard." This very potent drug is used intravenously for the palliative treatment of Hodgkin's disease and certain cancers. It's so powerful that the contraindications are many. More in keeping with mustard's traditional use as a plaster is *Musterole Deep Strength Rub*, available in gel, cream, or ointment form. Sad to say, the name *Musterole* is suggestive of mustard, but mustard is not one of its ingredients.

Bach flower remedies work on one's emotional state to improve one's physical state. They were developed in the late 1920s by English physician Edward Bach, M.B., B.S., D.P.H., who was looking for a better way to treat the mental distress his patients experienced. Remedy 21, Mustard, is formulated to relieve the type of depression that arrives for no apparent reason. The sunny yellow flowers of mustard signified "cheerfulness" in the eyes of Dr. Bach. He believed that the essence of mustard flowers would bring to the forefront whatever was causing feelings of depression, thus enabling the patient to deal with dark thoughts and banish them, so that cheerfulness was restored.

MUSTARD-BASED REMEDIES

Mustard has been used for centuries as a medicinal. Now you, too, can add it to your arsenal against colds and congestion, arthritic aches and pains, digestive disorders, and more. Following are Ayurvedic, Traditional Chinese Medicine, and other traditional recipes for treatments using mustard.

External Mustard Remedies

The most common use of mustard medicinally is in a plaster, or poultice. Because a mustard plaster is the first thing most people think of when considering mustard as a medicinal herb, this section starts off with a mustard plaster, as well as other time-honored external treatments. A plaster or poultice is composed of a soft substance that is mixed with water to form a paste. A cloth (cotton flannel is traditional) is placed on the skin of the affected area, and the paste is spread atop the cloth. The plaster is then overwrapped with another cloth to increase the effectiveness of the herb's properties.

A mustard plaster is used to increase blood flow to the area, thereby breaking up congestion, helping expel phlegm, relaxing stressed muscles, soothing aches, relieving painful joints, and easing inflammation. Mustard plasters have been used throughout recorded history to relieve backache and sciatica or to treat an "irritated" kidney. A mustard plaster can also help bring a stubborn boil to a head or open an abscess. Old-time healers also used mustard to draw out splinters and reduce the risk of infection. The increased blood flow caused by this rubefacient herb helps carry away toxins from the infected area.

The ancients used mustard poultices extensively. As recently as your great-grandmother's day, a mustard plaster was the first line of defense against lung congestion, bronchitis, and even pneumonia. Your great-grandfather doubtless appreciated the relief it brought to his arthritic joints and sore muscles, as well. If you want to experience mustard's medicinal magic yourself, here's how to prepare and use some external mustard remedies.

Mustard Plaster

Use a mortar and pestle (or seed grinder) to pulverize a quantity of mustard seeds. The amount of seeds you will need depends on the area to be treated. For most purposes, four to six ounces of seeds will be sufficient. If you don't want to follow the example of previous generations and grind your own seeds, four to six ounces of prepared mustard powder can be used in place of four to six ounces of ground seeds. It is available in most supermarkets. Remember that mustard is *very* hot. Most authorities say that the ground seed must be diluted so that it does not cause severe discomfort, as well as burning and blistering of the skin.

The majority of sources I consulted recommend mixing the mustard seed powder with varying amounts of linseed (flaxseed) meal or wheat flour. However, few households nowadays have linseed meal on hand. Both linseed meal and wheat flour will soften the action of the mustard without canceling out its important properties.

1. Mix one part ground mustard seed or powder with an equal amount of wheat flour. Dilute the mixture with sufficient cold water to achieve a soft paste. Add water slowly until the paste is thick, but not so stiff that it's difficult to work with. Aim for a soft, spreadable consistency.

2. Place a clean cloth large enough to cover the area to be treated on a clean, flat surface ready to receive the paste. Cotton flannel, linen, or several layers of muslin are good choices, but don't use thin cotton sheeting.

3. Apply the mustard paste to one side of the cloth, and fold another layer of cloth over the paste to completely enclose the herb. Remember that mustard is a hot herb. Contact with the skin may cause blistering and should be avoided.

4. Although mustard creates its own heat, to increase effectiveness and speed things up, you may warm the plaster to a temperature of between 104°F and 110°F by heating it for ten to fifteen seconds in a microwave.

5. When the plaster is ready, cleanse the area of the body to be treated by wiping it down with hydrogen peroxide to rid the surface of lingering bacteria. If the patient is a child or has sensitive skin, coating the area to be treated with a film of olive oil or a beaten egg white before applying the plaster is a time-honored sensible precaution.

6. Apply the plaster to the affected area. Overwrap the plaster with another clean cloth (wool is traditional) to hold in the heat and keep the patient's clothes and bedclothes clean. If necessary, you can use safety pins to secure the overwrap. If you wish, you may opt for plastic wrap as an overwrap instead of cotton flannel or wool.

7. Some areas of the body are more sensitive than others. For example, deep heat on an arthritic knee is more easily tolerated than on the more tender chest area. If the patient is comfortable, leave the plaster in place until the surface of the skin begins to redden and a burning sensation is felt. There will be a throbbing pain as the plaster draws out infection and neutralizes toxins. When the pain subsides, the plaster is spent and should be removed. Do not leave the plaster in place for longer than one hour.

8. After the plaster is removed, bathe the treated area with cool (not cold) water to stop the burn. Dry the area. Then finish up with a dusting of baby powder (your grandmother probably used flour or cornstarch) to soothe the skin. If the patient complains at any time during treatment, remove the plaster immediately and adhere to the instructions following the removal of the plaster.

Old-time herbalists believed that blistering of the skin signaled that toxins were being brought to the surface. They thought that toxins could be eliminated by lancing the blisters, but we now know that belief is outmoded. Without protection, mustard can blister the skin. Just remember that a comforting feeling of heat is good; intolerable burning is not.

Asian Mustard Compress

In Chinese medicine, as in Western medicine, a mustard compress (or plaster) is a favorite remedy for the common cold.

1. Mix equal parts mustard powder and water to form a plaster. Apply to the chest area and wrap a cloth over it.

2. Allow the compress to remain in place for about twenty minutes.

Because this compress is not cut with flour and the instructions say to apply the mixture directly on the skin, test its effect first on a small sensitive area of the body, such as the crook of your arm. Wait ten minutes for any reaction before applying to the chest area. The source I consulted stated that if the skin turns red, add flour to the mixture, and test it again.

This same remedy is used in Traditional Chinese Medicine against frostbite. The instructions say to use a cloth between the skin and the affected area, which is how mustard plasters are used in the West. With frostbite, mustard must not touch the skin directly, as it may deepen the frostbite.

Asian Knee Bath

I expect this remedy will work as well for other stiff and sore parts of the body, but the source I consulted called it a "knee bath." It is considered to be a premier treatment for knee pain.

1. Fill one-quarter of the bathtub with hot water.

2. Add $1^1/_2$ cups of yellow mustard powder to the bath, and swish it around with your hand until the powder dissolves.

3. Relax in the treated waters for fifteen minutes.

4. Shower off with cool water.

Asian Mustard Infusion

This remedy is said to be effective for arthritis or rheumatism in any part of the body.

1. Simmer together equal parts of mustard leaves, stems, seeds, and root for fifteen minutes in enough water to cover the part of the body to be treated. Strain.

2. When the mixture cools to a temperature that is hot but not intolerable, soak the affected area in the mustard-infused water until the water cools.

Asian Mustard Rub

In Chinese medicine, mustard and ginger are often used together. This rub is considered to be very effective in clearing the worst chest cold or the nastiest deep-seated cough. This warming rub works equally well on sore muscles and stiff, aching joints.

1. Combine 1 teaspoon dry mustard and 1 teaspoon dry ginger with 2 tablespoons sesame seed or olive oil. Test the mixture on the skin in the bend of the patient's arm to see if any irritation develops. Wait ten minutes before proceeding.

2. If all is well, rub the mixture directly on the patient's chest and back just before he or she goes to bed. Rub it in until a warmth and tingling is felt.

3. Have the patient put on an old tee shirt (the mixture will stain clothing) and enjoy a good night's sleep.

4. Wash the rub off in the morning, soaping well to remove any oil residue.

My sister, who is troubled with arthritic knees, likes this rub very much. She said the warmth penetrates well and is very comforting. The effect lasts about an hour before fading away.

Mustard and Ginger for Cold Feet

This very old Asian treatment is said to be a sure-cure for cold feet. It is believed that when this simple treatment is continued daily for a period of time, cold feet will become a thing of the past.

1. Mix 3 to 4 tablespoons of dry mustard with just enough juice expressed from fresh ginger root to make a smooth paste.

2. Apply the mixture to the soles of the feet, and put on a pair of thick socks. You should feel your feet heating up very quickly.

3. When the effect fades—in about an hour—wash the mixture off and put on a fresh pair of thick socks.

Ayurvedic Deep-Heat Rub

The following is a Vedic recipe for mustard massage oil. Caution: Never use mustard oil on mucous membranes, or anywhere near your eyes. It has the potential to cause blindness. This rub is good for sore muscles and stiff, aching joints, but do not use it for headaches.

1. Stir 1 tablespoon of cracked mustard seed into 4 tablespoons of sesame oil. The easiest way to crack mustard seeds is to put them into a large square of heavy aluminum foil, fold the square "envelope-style" over the seeds, and then pound it with a hammer. You'll be surprised at how tough these little seeds are.

2. Simmer this mixture over very low heat for 30 minutes. The oil will turn very dark in color.

3. Remove from heat, and strain the seeds from the oil. Allow the mixture to cool to a comfortable temperature before using.

Ayurvedic Mustard Infusion

Mustard is an effective analgesic and muscle relaxant that is said to quickly relieve muscle spasms. This infusion may also be used for the relief of joint pain.

1. To soak a small part of the body, such as a hand or a foot, put two tablespoons of cracked mustard seed (see above for instructions for cracking mustard seed) in the center of a small square of cloth. To soak a large area in a bathtub, use 6 tablespoons. Bring up the four corners of the cloth, then tie the packet "hobo-style."

2. Place the smaller bag of mustard in a basin of hot water and swish it around, or put the larger bag underneath running hot water in the bathtub.

3. Immerse the affected part of the body in the infusion until the warmth of this hot herb brings relief.

The British Footbath

A mustard footbath is a favorite in the United Kingdom and all over Europe as a treatment for headaches and a congested chest. It's considered a good preventive measure whenever a cold seems to be coming on, and it can also help relieve a chill. The drawing action of the herb will help bring blood to the lower part of the body, thereby relieving congestion of the head and lungs.

1. Dissolve $1/4$ cup of mustard-seed powder in one pint of freshly boiled water.

2. Put 3 cups of very warm water in a basin, and add the dissolved mustard-seed powder. Stir to blend.

3. Soak your feet in the hot mustard-infused water for at least 10 minutes, or until the water cools.

4. Dry your feet and put on a pair of warm socks or slippers.

Note: The English are particularly fond of mustard baths. So much so, in fact, that single bath-sized packets of a mustard powder formula mixed with other herbs, including eucalyptus, rosemary, wintergreen, and thyme, sell briskly, as does the 8-ounce tin of the same mustard formula. If you want to try this British import, you'll find out where to get it in the Resources section of this book. You may be interested to know that the same company that puts out Mustard Bath packets also offers a Mustard Rub, which consists of what is described as a "titillating" mustard oil for massage and deep-muscle therapy.

Mustard and Honey for Hemorrhoids

According to Traditional Chinese Medicine, this combination provides relief from the soreness and itching associated with hemorrhoids.

1. Mix equal parts of mild mustard powder and honey together until they form a well-mixed cream.

2. Apply to the affected area.

Mustard and Vinegar for Paralysis

This interesting, very old Asian remedy was once a therapy for those suffering from paralysis.

1. Mix equal parts of mild mustard powder and vinegar together.

2. Just before bedtime, apply the mixture to the paralyzed part of the body.

The directions for this therapy state that once the patient awakens from sleep, there should be a noticeable improvement in his or her ability to move.

Internal Mustard Remedies

Internally, mustard is often used in teas and other preparations as a digestive aid. You'll find that it can also be used to relieve chest congestion as well as a few other ailments. Here are some recipes for internal mustard remedies.

Constipation Remedy

Mustard has been used to treat constipation for centuries. This herb works slowly but surely. It relieves constipation naturally by encouraging peristalsis, the rhythmic motion that initiates a bowel movement.

1. Mix $^1/_2$ teaspoon of freshly ground mustard seed (see directions for grinding seeds on page 37) or mustard powder in $^1/_2$ cup of cool water.

2. Drink the mixture on an empty stomach first thing in the morning for two days. You may have your breakfast after drinking this remedy.

Congee

This recipe is very ancient. This particular congee is prescribed for deep cough, chest congestion, chronic bronchitis, and asthma. It is said to sweep away phlegm, warm the core of the body, aid the stomach, and promote urination.

Stir 1 cup of washed and finely chopped mustard greens and 2 cups of uncooked rice into 10 cups of pure spring water. (Do not use tap water—the chemicals, such as chlorine, used to kill the bacteria in the water will change the properties of the congee.) Slowly simmer the mixture until the rice and greens become indivisible from the water—about 3 to 4 hours. Some of the water will evaporate, but the end result will be a very thin watery gruel. The ancients simmered congee in a kettle on the stove for hours, presumably stirring occasionally. If you have a Crock-Pot, set it at low setting, and let the congee cook overnight.

If you are interested in learning more about this fascinating little-known adjunct to Chinese medicine, consult *The Book of Jook: Chinese Medicinal Porridges* by Bob Flaws.

Digestible Vegetables

Mustard is traditionally used in Ayurvedic medicine to relieve or prevent indigestion. To improve the digestibility of vegetables, the good cooks of India follow the ancient teachings. It has long been believed that cooking with mustard seed makes vegetables very light and easy to digest. Here's how it's done. The proportions are not critical.

1. Heat 2 tablespoons of sesame oil in a pan. When the oil is hot, add 2 pinches of mustard seed. Stir until the seeds pop.

2. Add $1/4$ cup onion cut into thin slices and 2 crushed cloves of garlic. Stir to coat the onion and garlic with the oil mixture.

3. Cut the vegetables of your choice into small pieces, and add them to the oil.

4. Cook, stirring constantly, until the vegetables are tender-crisp.

Digestive and Diuretic Tea

This infusion comes from herbalist A.I. Coffin (1798–1866), who himself received it from Samuel Thomason (1769–1843), who was a noted authority on American Indian herbs and their uses. Thomason taught what he called Physio-Medicalism, a protocol that focused on the use of herbs for body correction. Although he was later credited with many amazing discoveries, Dr. Thomason was persecuted by the medical professionals of his day.

1. Combine $1/2$ ounce of cracked mustard seeds with one ounce of fresh horseradish root, sliced.

2. Add the herbs to 8 ounces of freshly boiled water.

3. Cover and let stand in a covered vessel for 4 hours. Strain.

4. Take 3 tablespoonsful three times daily.

This remedy is useful in the treatment of water retention and edema. However, sudden or abnormal fluid retention may be a sign of a serious illness. Heart disease, kidney disease, and liver dysfunction may cause fluid accumulation. These conditions should not be self-treated. Any abnormal fluid retention should be brought to the attention of your doctor.

Hiccup Cure

One old herbal book that I consulted assured me that mustard "floure" is a sure-cure for stubborn "hiccoughs." If you want to try it, here's what to do:

1. Dissolve $1/2$ teaspoonful of mustard flour in a teacupful of freshly boiled water.

2. Drink it all down as soon as you can without burning your mouth.

3. If needed, the treatment may be repeated in 10 minutes.

Respiratory and Digestive Distress Tea

Mustard tea acts as an expectorant by stimulating the flow of fluids, thereby thinning mucus, making it easier to expel. Mustard is also said to help the digestive process by causing an increased flow of digestive juices. This herb is sometimes used to stimulate a flagging appetite. It also acts as a mild diuretic and is said to help in cases of delayed menstruation.

1. Make a decoction of mustard seed by putting 1 teaspoon of seed in 8 ounces of freshly boiled water. Cover and let the mixture steep for 20 minutes, then strain the seeds.

2. Drink up to 3 cups of tea per day for up to 3 weeks, as needed.

This tea is very pale in color and very mild in taste. Do not be deceived. Even though you may not notice the bite or the warmth while sipping it, it works very effectively internally. You will feel a warming effect in your stomach and notice a bit of heat in the aftertaste.

Remedy for a Stuffy Nose

You won't find this home remedy in any book I know of, except this one. This is something my family has found helpful for at least a couple of generations. It's wonderful for opening up a stuffy nose and clogged sinuses, and it's my personal favorite.

1. Heap thinly sliced raw onions on thinly sliced rye bread.

2. Slather on the hottest mustard you have on hand. I use horseradish or chipotle mustard or mix up dry mustard powder especially for the occasion.

3. Savor the sandwich.

I think this sandwich is so good, it's worth suffering a cold to eat it. I don't know why I never fix this sandwich unless I have a stuffy nose, but I don't. I must be programmed by generations of treatments to regard this delight as "medicine," I guess.

In the next chapter, I'll let you in on some surprising uses scientists have found for this amazing herb.

4

Mustard Miscellany

"Unimportant, of course, I meant," the King hastily said, and went on to himself in an undertone, "important— unimportant—unimportant—important," as if he were trying to decide which word sounded best.

—*Alice in Wonderland*
Lewis Carroll (1832–1898)

While I was doing research on mustard in preparation for writing this book, I started out by conducting a search of all existing scientific literature on mustard. What I received was an overwhelming 120 pages listing abstracts (short summaries) of published papers. Each of the 120 pages contained from eight to twelve abstracts, meaning that there have been at least 1,000 studies on this ancient golden herb. I was thrilled! Several of the abstracts were very old or not useful; nonetheless, I discovered quite a few fascinating uses for mustard in these pages.

This is a very interesting chapter. Quite simply, it contains a wealth of the delicious "unimportant" minutia on mustard I uncovered during my research for this book, as well as one very *important* use for the mustard plant. It's called phytoremediation, and I'll tell you all about it a little later on. I think you'll be amazed at what scientists around the world have discovered that mustard can do. Here's a sampling of the interesting tidbits I unearthed.

USING MUSTARD AS A PRESERVATIVE

In addition to mustard's positive effects in the body, mustard has also been found to be an effective preservative for foods and drinks. Read on to learn more.

Preserving Wine With Mustard

Would you believe that wine could be stabilized by using a bit of mustard? Apparently, it works. In 1961, Drs. D.K. Chalenko and T.F. Korsakova of Moscow published a study entitled, "Methods of Stabilization of Semi-Sweet Wines." According to the abstract, the European and Slavic wines tested were Riesling, Kaberne, Pukhlyakovskii, Hungarian Muscatel, and Aligote. The scientists used 0.4 grams of mustard per liter of wine. "Semi-sweet wines [stabilized with mustard] had high taste and aroma qualities and were almost identical in this respect to wines prepared by the classical procedure," the study said. "These semi-sweet wines can be recommended for commercial production."

While the scientists who conducted this study may have recommended this method for the preservation of wines, I have yet to see any wine that has been stabilized this way. Most wines are still preserved with sulfites.

Preserving Fruit Juices With Mustard

If you prefer a nonalcoholic beverage, you should be interested to learn that the above procedure also works with fruit juices. In a 1949 research paper entitled "Mustard as a Preservative for Fruit Juices," O. Kosker, Carl R. Fellers, and W.B. Esselen, Jr., reported that "The addition of 11 to 22 ppm (parts per million) of mustard oil or its equivalent in ground mustard to fresh apple or grape juices exerted a preservative action in retarding fermentation."

Preserving Meat and Fish With Mustard

If you like mustard on your roast beef, as I do, you'll appreciate this section. In 1951, G.B. Dubrova, N.I. Kovalev, and M.S. Osmolovskaya of the Leningrad Soviet Trade Institute published their research entitled "Experimental Storage of Meat in Mustard." They reported that storing raw meat in a "mustard solution" in airtight containers at room temperature prevented spoilage for up to 144 hours. However, the report concluded with this note, "Meat steeped in mustard solution could be kept about 48 hours [and then eaten], but after 144 hours the taste properties made it unsuitable for consumption." In other words, mustard prevented the meat from spoiling, but after sitting in a mustard solution for six days, the meat had such a strong mustard flavor that it was unpalatable. I really love the characteristic smell, flavor, heat, and bite of good mustard, but I think meat steeped for 144 hours in a mustard solution would be much too much of a good thing.

In 1958, I.S. Zagaevskil published a paper entitled, "Use of Levomycetin, Phthalazol, and Mustard Powder for Preserving Meat Products, Tripe, and Fish." Chemical preservatives such as levomycetin and phthalazol have been around a very long time, but mustard has been around even longer. Dr. Zagaevskil reported that "A combination of levomycetin with phthalazol intensifies the bacteriostatic and in part the bactericidal action . . . in regard to microorganisms causing spoilage of tripe [stomach], meat products, and fish. . . . The storage period of refrigerated products and fish is doubled by storing with crushed ice containing a concentration of 5 percent mustard powder."

Preserving Bread With Mustard

In 1958, A.Z. Kamaletdinov published a report on his research in a paper entitled "The Preservation of Bread to be Used by Mountain Climbers." In this study, Dr. Kamaletdinov investigated "the possibility of preserving bread with table mustard or medicinal mustard preparations." According to the results of this study, "Bread can be preserved for up to two months by covering its surface, or the paper used for wrapping, with a thin layer of either [medicinal mustard preparations or table] mustard, and then wrapping in two layers of waxed paper." Apparently, man cannot live on a mountaintop on bread alone. It seems we also need mustard.

Preserving Root Vegetables With Mustard

A.I. Grinum of the Leningrad Institute published a paper entitled "Use of Antiseptics and Antibiotics During Storage of Carrots," in 1959. Mustard was among several antiseptic substances used in this study. Carrots were combined with the antiseptic substances and then stored in baskets containing sand or wood shavings. The carrots then were left undisturbed for 160 days in the sand, or 55 days in the shavings. At the close of the study, 92 percent of the carrots protected by the pulverized mustard were judged to be of acceptable quality, whether they were stored in sand or wood shavings. If you're planning to spend a few years in an isolated cabin somewhere, take along a goodly supply of powdered mustard. This treatment would probably work equally well on all root vegetables, including potatoes.

USING MUSTARD TO COMBAT THE OXIDATION OF FATS

Fats are particularly susceptible to the chemical process of oxidation, which causes them to turn rancid. Mustard has been found to be effective at preventing the oxidation of fats. Here's a report on yet another study from the former Union of Soviet Socialist Republics, entitled "Natural Additives—Stabilizers of Fat in Food Concentrates." L.A. Fomicheva, et al., of the Moscow Technological Institute did the work in 1986. The paper states, "Of 23 natural additives, mustard powder, soybean flour, carrot, red pepper, coriander, and horseradish were more effective as antioxidants with respect to confectionery fat peroxidation [fats in sweets turning rancid] than was the chemical antioxidant Na [sodium] glutamate. . . . Mustard powder was most effective; no peroxide compounds were detected in fats that were treated with mustard powder at 45 degrees and then solidified and maintained at room temperature for ten months." In other words, the fats treated with mustard powder showed no signs of turning rancid.

An earlier study by the Japanese also documented the antioxidant properties of mustard oil and suggested its use as a fat preservative. In a 1982 study entitled "Mustard Oil Glycosides as Food Antioxidants," K.K. Wasaki Kinjirushi pointed out that organic compounds in mustard oil called glycosides are "antioxidants for foods rich in oils and fats."

USING MUSTARD AS AN ANTIBACTERIAL AGENT

In 1943, the *Fruit Products Journal* published an article entitled "Spice Oils and Their Components for Controlling Microbial Surface Growth," written by H.B. Blum and F.W. Fabian. These researchers subjected several bacteria (*Acetobacter, Saccharomyces, Cerevisiae,* and *Mycoderma*) to oil extracted from several spices, including mustard seed, cinnamon, cassia, and cloves. It was determined that mighty mustard has greater antimicrobial actions than the other spices that were tested. The study concludes, "The germicidal value of a spice is due to an active germicidal principle present in the spice. . . . The relative effectiveness for the spice oils was not the same for all tests and organisms. However, oil of mustard was consistently superior to the others."

USING MUSTARD AS AN ACNE TREATMENT

Are you interested in a primarily natural treatment that works against acne? John R. King applied for a U.S. patent in 1982 for just such a remedy. The article accompanying the application was entitled "Composition for Treating Acne." The ingredient list for this potion included such items as mustard seeds, raw oats, zinc gluconate, brewer's yeast, egg yolks, peroxide, alcohol, and chemical preservatives. Dr. King said, "Test results indicated a resolution of acne [anywhere] from 75 to 100 percent." This "recipe" sounds almost good enough to eat.

USING MUSTARD AS A HAIR TREATMENT

Here's another interesting formula. In 1977, William L. Vinson applied for a patent for a "Hair Pressing Composition" composed of "a petroleum base, lanolin, coconut oil, and an effective amount of weeping willow extract, and extracts from mustard greens and corn with other optional ingredients such as glycerol, vinegar, and wheat germ oil." Dr. Vinson's composition is meant to "curl straight hair or straighten kinky hair."

USING MUSTARD FOR URANIUM DETECTION

If you're planning on prospecting for uranium the next time you're in Colorado, here's a report on a fascinating study published in the *U.S. Geological Survey Bulletin* 1085-A in 1960. This report, authored by Helen L. Cannon, is entitled "The Development of Botanical Methods of Prospecting for Uranium on the Colorado Plateau." It seems that mustard has an affinity for uranium, so wild mustard tends to grow in areas of uranium deposits. This makes mustard effective as an indicator plant for uranium—its growth can signal the presence of uranium deposits. Uranium can also be detected by analysis of samples from deep-rooted trees. The study concludes with this advice: "The most useful indicator plants are loco weed and plants of the mustard family."

This leads us to the most exciting, and certainly most important, piece in this chapter—phytoremediation.

Mustard Gas

Although mustard has been proposed as the primary ingredient in self-defense sprays, mustard gas itself is not derived from mustard seed. Nonetheless, because of its mustardlike effects and similar composition, the gas will forever be known as mustard gas. Mustard got a bad reputation in World War I when the Germans introduced mustard gas as a chemical warfare agent. Chemical agents, especially those that burn and start secondary fires, are of ancient origin. Smoke and stenches, mainly from sulfur compounds, were used as a defense in ancient times; however, the Germans turned those early efforts into a science.

Mustard gas comes from a light, colorless, oily liquid composed of carbon, hydrogen, sulfur, and chlorine. The vapor attacks the mucous membranes of the respiratory tract, destroys lung tissue, and blisters the skin. For those unlucky enough to be on the field when the gas came in, the effects included internal and external burns, blindness, and in some cases, death.

From 1915 to 1918, the Germans introduced a succession of poison gases, which were quickly duplicated by the Allies. In 1915, the Germans began the competition by using chlorine gas. The Allies promptly developed gas masks and also began producing chlorine. Next the Germans introduced phosgene, another type of poisonous gas. The allies then improved their gas masks and also began producing phosgene. It was in 1917 that the Germans began using mustard gas, and by 1918, the toxic gas was in widespread use by both sides. After 1918, the opposition to the use of chemicals in warfare was so strong that they were outlawed.

Volatile chemicals may have been banned as weapons of war, but, in milder form, they are used nowadays for self-defense. In 1975, a Japanese scientist by the name of Tatsuo Enomoto applied for a patent for an "Aerosol Agent for Self-Defense Use," which was the predecessor of pepper spray. This is where mustard enters the equation. Enomoto recommended the use of extracts from *Capsicum* (hot pepper seed), *Brassica nigra* (black mustard seed), or *Sinapis alba* (white mustard seed) as the active ingredients in a spray designed for defense. The conclusion to the paper states, "The mixture was filled in aerosol cans for self-defense use. The preparation proved highly irritant, but was incombustible and nontoxic."

USING MUSTARD FOR PHYTOREMEDIATION

Phytoremediation is the use of plants to leach heavy metal contaminants from soil. I stumbled upon this use for mustard quite by accident. During the time that I was writing this book, I read a one-paragraph account in a local newspaper that mentioned briefly that mustard was being used to clean up a lead-contaminated site in New Jersey where batteries had once been manufactured. In an attempt to learn more about this, I contacted the Department of Site Remediation for the State of New Jersey, which directed me to Michael Blaylock, Ph.D., of Phytotech, Incorporated, the company in charge of the cleanup of the site. Dr. Blaylock was very helpful as he patiently answered my questions.

It was mustard's efficiency as an indicator plant that led to its use for cleaning up toxic contamination in what are known as "brownfields"—sites contaminated by heavy metals. Here's the progression of events. In the early 1990s, a scientist named Ilya Raskin, who was then a professor of plant biology at Rutgers University, read several papers written by Russian researchers in the 1930s and '40s promoting the use of indicator plants such as mustard to locate rich underground deposits of metals. The Russian scientists showed that large stands of indicator plants could be used to identify areas that could be profitably mined. In one of those stunning events that may yet change the way the world deals with polluted land and water, Raskin decided to investigate plants that absorb metals with an eye to using them to absorb toxins from contaminated sites. It took a number of years of exhaustive research with various plant species, but Raskin and his coworkers at Rutgers succeeded.

It turns out that *Brassica juncea*, common brown mustard, is the champion at sucking lead, chromium, cadmium, zinc, and copper from the soil. Brown mustard can also be used to control selenium levels on croplands where this metal is too high to bear healthy foodstuffs for human consumption. Yes, there is increasing research showing that the body needs selenium, but no more than 200 micrograms daily. Amounts greater than this can cause serious health problems.

In 1993, when the basic research on the absorptive powers of the various plants was concluded, Rutgers University helped establish a New Jersey company called Phytotech to carry on with the research and put this new technology into practice. In the United States alone, there are around 30,000 sites that are contaminated with toxins. Phytotech is cleaning up some of them with three important types of phytoremediation called phytoextraction, phytostabilization, and rhizofiltration. Phytoextraction is the use of the roots and aboveground shoots of metal-accumulating plants to transport and concentrate metals from the soil. Phytostabilization is the use of plants to prevent toxic metals in soil from being absorbed by crops and from seeping into ground water, thus preventing toxins from entering into the food chain. Brown mustard has proven to be the best choice for both of these technologies. Rhizofiltration is the use of plant roots to separate, absorb, and concentrate toxic metals from polluted aqueous streams. Mustard is often used in this technology.

One huge advantage that mustard brings to the phytoremediation process is that it reaches maturity and can be harvested so quickly that it's possible to grow three crops on the same site during a single growing season. Although mustard has documented power in the decontamination department, Phytotech has developed additional soil additives that make the toxins more easily absorbed by the plants, which enables the mustard to leach out even more toxins from the soil than it can do on its own.

Although a few other companies are involved in phytoremediation, Phytotech is the pioneer in the field and has the most brownfield sites under cultivation. In a Boston neighborhood, Phytotech has sowed three plantings of mustard, which has leached as much as 45 percent of the excess lead out of a seriously contaminated plot. In Trenton, New Jersey, Phytotech is growing mustard on a brownfield site where batteries were once manufactured. This site, named "Magic Marker" because it was purchased by that company, was once heavily contaminated with lead. In one growing season, Phytotech has documented a reduction in lead to levels within the legal safety limits of 400 parts per million in 70 percent of the areas where mustard was grown. A chromium-contaminated site near Liberty State Park in New Jersey is also getting the mustard treatment. Phytotech has even had success using brown mustard to remove radionuclides (disintegrated atoms left behind by the emission of electromagnetic nuclear radiation), including cesium-137 and strontium-90, from the soil at a site in Chernobyl, the Ukranian city that was the site of a major nuclear power plant accident. A site in Ashtabula, Ohio, that was heavily contaminated with uranium is getting the same treatment.

Over a five-year period, cleanup costs of common toxins are estimated at $34 billion, and neutralizing radioactive contamination is estimated at $200 billion. Current treatments for soils contaminated with toxic metals include fixation, landfilling, and leaching. Fixation involves the chemical processing of soils to prevent metals from entering the ground water. After the chemicals have done their work, the surface soil must be treated to eliminate penetration by water to ensure that rainwater does not percolate through the soil and carry any leftover toxins into the ground water. Another cleanup process is landfilling. The government permits the excavation, transport, and deposit of contaminated soil in a hazardous waste landfill. The leaching process uses acid solutions or proprietary chemicals to remove certain metals from soil. This process can be effective in cleaning soil.

Phytoremediation has notable advantages over other methods of soil decontamination. While it does take longer to grow a series of crops on a contaminated site than it does to employ other technologies, the cost of growing the crops is less overall and it's environmentally safe. Phytoremediation is estimated to be between 25 to 50 percent more effective than traditional permanent remediation technologies. See Table 4.1 below.

Phytoremediation provides an environmentally safe means of removing contaminants that is preferable to the current method of

Table 4.1. Phytoremediation vs. Other Technologies

Treatment	Cost per Cubic Meter	Time Required	Additional Expenses	Safety Issues
Phytoremediation	$15–40	18–60 months	Time, Land commitment	Residue disposal
Fixation	$90–200	6–9 months	Excavation and transport, Long-term monitoring	Contaminants can leach into ground water
Landfills	$100–400	6–9 months	Long-term monitoring	Contaminants can leach into ground water
Soil extraction; Leaching	$250–500	8–12 months	These processes are only practical if done on a site of a minimum of 5,000 cubic meters; Chemical recycling	Residue disposal

Mustard Uses That Didn't Quite Cut the Mustard

Since mustard is so effective in so many ways, scientists decided to test its effectiveness as a mosquito repellent. In 1960, the University of Manitoba in Canada released a report written by A.J. Thorsteinson entitled "Olfactory Responses of Mosquito and Stable Flies to Some Natural Chemicals." Dr. Thorsteinson reports that "of a number of fatty acids investigated for repellency to stable flies, pelargonic acid [from geraniums] was the most effective. . . . Extracts of lilac and strawberry . . . were also repellent."

I'm sorry to have to tell you that my personal favorite, mustard, didn't make the grade. The report says that, "The odors of sweet clover and mustard blossoms attracted mosquitoes. . . ." If you have a cabin by a shallow lake, keep your patch of mustard greens well away from the water and mow down the sweet clover. Mosquitoes favor marshland as a breeding ground, as you probably know. There's no sense scenting the area with the perfume that attracts them.

Mustard has also been considered for use as a polishing agent. A.I. Tatarenkov applied for a patent in the former U.S.S.R. in 1966 for a "Paste for Polishing and Grinding of Parts," which consisted of, among other things, an abrasive powder and mustard.

I think Dr. Tatarenkov has hit on something that qualifies as a household hint. I tried his idea out on one of my old dark and dingy copper-bottomed pots by using plain scouring powder, which qualifies as an abrasive, on one half and scouring powder mixed with a grainy brown prepared mustard on the other half. I got a good shine on both halves, but I didn't have to work nearly as hard on the area where I had applied the mustard mixture. When I tried using mustard powder along with the scouring powder, it worked even better. I should tell you that I don't display my pots and pans, and I don't really care if the copper bottoms get scratched, either from banging them on the stove or from an abrasive. If you have beautiful copper pieces that you display, don't try this idea. Copper needs gentle cleaning.

removing contaminated soil and disposing of it in landfills where it can cause future problems. Getting rid of the toxin-contaminated plants after harvest is quickly accomplished by burning them. The ash contains the contaminants, but the contaminants are concentrated into a much smaller mass that can be disposed of economically. It's even possible to extract the leftover metals and recycle them.

If the problem is heavy metal contamination of water, precipitation (also called flocculation), ion exchange, reverse osmosis, and microfiltration processes are used. Precipitation is a process that uses chemicals to concentrate toxins into a mass that can be removed. Unfortunately, the special characteristics of certain toxic metals make precipation difficult and expensive. A recently developed ion-exchange process assumes that the metal can be separated from the water and recovered from the residue for disposal. Reverse osmosis uses a microfiltration system that catches toxins. It is widely used to purify seawater for drinking in arid countries, and is used by some companies that supply bottled drinking water in the United States. This technology is effective, but, in purifying sea water, it creates a salty residue. This process is also relatively expensive. Precipitation and microfiltration can be used, for example, to recover radionuclides from water, but are very costly. Rhizofiltration offers the same obvious advantages over current methods of cleaning water as phytoremediation does for soil cleanup.

In fact, the use of plants to decontaminate soil and water is so important that the EPA's Bioremediation Action Committee and international environmental agencies are working to ensure that the benefits of phytoremediation will be considered when plans are made to clean up a site. I find it very satisfying to learn that—given a little help—Mother Nature can cleanse the planet of many of the toxic pollutants mankind has visited on the Earth, and I am thrilled to know that mustard is the first choice of the phytoremediation experts.

Considering all you've learned in this chapter about mustard's importance to the planet, I expect you to accord this golden herb the respect it deserves from now on! In the next chapter, we will take a look at mustard's importance outside of this planet, as we explore mustard's role in the supernatural.

5

Mustard and the Supernatural

It is indeed possible to live without mustard.
It's also possible to survive without music, poetry,
or art—possible but not much fun.

—Barry Levenson

Mustard has long played a role in the supernatural. Because it symbolizes many different things for many different cultures, it has been used in magic and has been recognized as a symbol in dreams and astrology for centuries.

MUSTARD AND DREAMS

Dreams are successions of images unreeled by the subconscious while we are sleeping. Most dream interpreters believe that what we dream is tied to the concerns we have when awake. In fact, dream analysis is a tool sometimes used in psychology in an attempt to tap into the unconscious mind. Many books have been written that link certain symbols that appear in dreams with emotions or events being thought or felt in the subconscious. Here's what some dream analysts say about mustard.

The mustard seed is a powerful and enduring symbol of faith. If you dream of mustard in any guise—be it the whole plant, the fresh green leaves, the fiery seeds, or even the root—dream interpreters say it indicates that you have faith that all things are possible. Dreaming of mustard in any form means you can look forward to receiving good news as a result of groundwork laid down by your fruitful efforts.

If you dream of eating mustard seeds and actually feel the fire in your mouth, it signifies that you have done something for which you are now sorry. An ill-considered act or some thoughtless words may have caused someone to suffer, and you are suffering because of it. The heat from the seeds indicates that you accept punishment and wish to atone for your wrongdoing. Go forward and make amends. Have faith that all will be well, and it will be.

Dreaming of eating unripe green mustard seeds before the time of harvest shows impatience and an inability to wait for good things to come to you. A person who has such dreams has a tendency to desire instant gratification, rather than to wait for something better. Another interpretation of the same dream says that the greedy early eating of the immature seed without thought of what may transpire later as a consequence shows the lavish waste of good fortune. Whether the good fortune that was wasted is health or wealth, this dreamer is under a heavy strain.

If a farmer were to dream of a meadow full of sunny yellow flowers and tender green leaves of mustard, this is said to be a sure sign of a successful crop and imminent joy. If a seafarer were to have this type of a dream, he or she would be assured of a successful voyage, with wealth at the end of it.

MUSTARD AND MAGIC

In almost all ancient cultures, religion and magic were intertwined. Then, as now, the tiny mustard seed was a symbol of perfect faith. The term "magic" itself is derived from the word *magi*, members of a priestly caste of ancient Persia who reputedly had magic powers.

Magic is the practice of using various techniques, including rites, spells, incantations, potions, charms, and amulets to produce supernatural effects. Those who practice the ancient forms of magic attempt to harness the mysterious forces of the universe to gain control over natural events.

The members of the societies of yesterday commonly relied on charms and amulets to attract good fortune and ward off evil. They engaged in stylized religious rites to honor the gods and ensure a bountiful harvest. Priests chanted incantations designed to placate an angry god who was withholding rain during a drought. Just about everyone brought gifts to the idols that were representations of various gods when seeking a special boon. Charms to bring back a lover who had strayed, or a charm bag to insure faithfulness in one's mate, were always in demand. The childless wore fertility charms and petitioned the heavens for a child.

Charm bags were also commonly known as conjure bags, medicine bags, gris-gris bags, mojo bags, hoodoo bags, or wanga bags. Whatever name they were called, the bags were usually handcut squares of soft cloth or soft well-worked leather. Magical objects thought to be imbued with special powers were placed in the square, the four ends of the square were drawn up, and a thin piece of leather was tied around the neck of the cloth "hobo-style" to keep the objects in place. The little charm bag was then worn on a thong around the neck or hung in a strategic place in the home or workplace.

Legend has it that with the right "magic" ingredients in the charm bag, a person's objective was assured, and he or she would live a long and fortunate life, as long as he or she was worthy. Mustard seeds were often the primary ingredient in certain specialized charm bags. Herbs and colored feathers were also common ingredients. Sometimes the substances were moistened with oil or mixed with a paste of water and flour, and formed into a ball and then placed in a charm bag. It is written that the number of objects in the bag must never total an even number.

Just for fun, what follows is a sampling of some old formulas once believed to create a powerful aura of good vibrations, thus insuring you would receive your heart's desire.

For Spiritual Blessings

It is written that when soliciting spiritual blessings, you need to use a combination of mustard seed, blessed thistle, and holy oil. A charm bag containing these three once-sacred ingredients was historically considered a fail-safe method of insuring the favorable attention of the gods.

To Insure Faithfulness From a Lover

To make sure that lovers remain faithful to one another, it is said that each should wear a bag that holds mustard seed, a red feather (red symbolizes love), lavender, vervain, and khus-khus. Khus-

khus, also called vetiver, is a grass grown in India whose roots yield a scented oil used in perfumery.

For Riches

If wealth and riches are on your wish-list, the ingredients to use are mustard seed, goldenseal, and a golden-yellow feather (yellow and gold relate to money).

For Protection

From old Mexico comes a legendary formula said to be a shield against evil and protection from danger. Prepare and wear a charm bag containing mustard seed, one pin, and a medallion of St. Barbara. St. Barbara was a second-century martyr who was killed for following the teachings of Christ at a time when Christians were considered heretics.

For Good Fortune in All Things

For an all-purpose wish bag, the formula is nine mustard seeds, one rabbit's foot, five new hardware nails, thirteen pences, and sacred bark. Once the bag is prepared, anoint it with sweet oil (or your personal fragrance) and rub it between your palms as you make your wish. To keep the "magic" strong, be sure to anoint the bag every seventh day with oil or fragrance.

For Mental Clarity

To enhance your mental powers and improve memory and recall of past events, wear a bag containing mustard seed, rosemary, and a blue feather (blue calms a restless spirit).

For Serenity

For an easy life, wear a charm bag containing mustard seed, clover, and a green feather (green is the serene color of nature). This charm was not meant to bring a life of ease and wealth, but rather a life devoid of problems.

For Protection Against Sorcery

In medieval times, mustard seeds were believed to have the power to protect against sorcery. Those who feared that black magic was being used against them buried mustard seeds deep under the front doorstep to prevent evil spirits from entering. For additional protection while sleeping, fearful people mixed equal amounts of mustard and flaxseeds and placed them in a blue bowl on one side of the bed, then placed cold water in a white bowl on the other side of the bed. Thus protected from evil influences, the superstitious slept easy.

To Identify Witches and Warlocks

Here's another legendary use for "magical" mustard seed. To unmask a witch or warlock hiding his or her identity, light a single candle in a dark room. Drop seven mustard seeds one by one into a small basin of water, all the while intoning the suspect's name. Watch out! If a shadowy shape appears to form in the water, it's a sure sign the person in question is guilty of practicing black art.

MUSTARD AND ASTROLOGY

It's very interesting to learn that many astrologers believe that various herbs are associated with particular planets. For example, the mustard plant is said to be in harmony with the planet Mars, which rules the zodiacal sign of Aries (March 21–April 20). That's why charms containing mustard seed are considered especially powerful when used by one born under the Sign of the Ram.

If you were born under another planetary influence, not to worry. Mustard is also reported to have an affinity for Tuesday. Its "magic" is enhanced when it is used on that day of the week. Mustard is also associated astrologically with the element fire—a reference, no doubt, to this herb's heat. Early Hindus reportedly used mustard seed to travel through the air, but the magic spell required to become airborne via mustard seed is long lost, if indeed it ever existed.

In one early European flower calendar, June 18th was the date assigned to the mustard flower. In the language of flowers, however, mustard signifies indifference. If you're sending flowers to someone you care about to celebrate a June 18th birthday, don't send mustard.

In the next chapter, let's return to the basic theme of this book with a look at the many mustard varieties available for your joy and delight.

6

Mustard Varieties

*I followed them into the kitchen and started going through
her cabinets as if assuming I'd find a cupful of .22 bullets....
For someone who was close to broke, Bonnie was spending
too much money on mustard: honey mustard, tarragon
mustard, green peppercorn mustard. I looked over at her.
Maybe I'd try a little mustard humor, clear the air....*

—*Magic Hour*
Susan Isaacs

Mustard is a favorite condiment in my household. I keep a
selection of mustard seeds on hand, including the tiny
black, the fat yellow, and the pale round seed varieties that
I use in various ways. I also routinely stock dry mustard powder
that I mix up when we order Chinese food. The restaurant never
seems to provide enough for us. Dry mustard powder is also essential in certain dishes that the whole family enjoys. You'll find recipes
for mustard creams and recipes that use mustard powder and
creams in Part Two.

I have one shelf on the door of my refrigerator devoted to prepared mustard. To please my family, I always have a stock of basic
mustard. For example, there's always someone who wants nothing
but plain yellow mustard, while someone else wants hearty coarse-
ground spicy brown deli-style mustard, and claims nothing else will
do. There are also those among us who favor honey mustard, and,
of course, Dijon mustard always gets a lot of votes, as do the hot
mustards with horseradish and/or chipotle peppers. You'll also find

jars of some of my new favorites—cranberry mustard, garlic mustard, tomato-basil mustard, orange and honey mustard, and tarragon mustard—tucked in among the old favorites that claim pride of place in my refrigerator. In fact, when I read *Magic Hour* by Susan Isaacs, from which I took the quote that opens this chapter, I bought some green peppercorn mustard and discovered I liked it very much.

I hope to encourage you to sample some new varieties of mustard the next time you're doing your marketing. In one of the supermarkets in which I shop, I counted fifty-three types of mustards. In another, I counted fifty-eight. Specialty and gourmet shops, as well as specialty and cooking catalogs offer many more varieties of mustard than the average supermarket does.

The section that follows includes many varieties of mustard. It by no means encompasses all the types of mustards available, but if you're a mustard aficionado, you'll enjoy identifying old favorites, and you're sure to discover some new varieties you'll be eager to sample, as I have. There are so many interesting flavors that I'm betting you'll find a few that will catch your fancy.

It's difficult, if not impossible, to try to describe how something tastes. What seems too hot for me, for example, may seem positively mild to someone else. I like grainy mustards, especially those smoothed with spirits, but my grandson calls them "yucky." Sweet, mild mustards please me, while some members of my family call my favorite fruity mustards "sickeningly sweet." In the end, you will have to do your own taste-test and make your own determination. I suggest that you use this chapter as a starting point. I bet you'll find your mouth watering. I start with a listing of basic mustards that I believe belongs in any well-stocked kitchen, followed by a variety of mustards grouped into categories.

BASIC MUSTARDS

If you have a selection of these basic mustards on hand, you're ready for anything. Any of the recipes included in this book can be made with any of the basic mustards, or you can choose among your personal favorites and use that one in a recipe. If you're relatively new to mustards, start with these, and branch out when you begin to feel adventurous.

Mustard Seed

Used whole, mustard seeds are crunchy and mild, with only a slight bite and just a bit of heat. You won't believe how good whole mustard seeds are on a sandwich until you try it. And, if you're going to make your own mustard from scratch, this is where to start. When ground and mixed with an equal amount of cold water, the flavor bursts through.

Dry Mustard Powder

Dry mustard powder lasts indefinitely. For a quick Chinese-style mustard, mix dry mustard powder with an equal amount of cold water, and let it sit for ten minutes. This mixture is guaranteed to clear your sinuses. Dry mustard powder is also called for in many recipes.

Deli-Style Mustard

Deli mustards are usually grainy but slightly mild. These mustards add a hint of mustard's pungent flavor to a sandwich or anything else without burning your mouth.

Dijon Mustard

The famous French-style mustards of America are made with white wine. They are assertive without being overpowering. Choose smooth or whole-grain for true mustard flavor enhanced with wine.

Stone-Ground and Whole-Grain Mustards

These mustards have a grainy texture with flecks of mustard seed. They are strong and pungent without being bitter. Expect true undiluted mustard flavor with some heat.

Yellow "Ballpark" Mustard

This mustard was everyone's favorite in childhood and still seems to please many people. If you have room for only one mustard in your refrigerator, this is the universal mustard that's welcomed by everyone.

SWEET MUSTARDS

All sweet mustards, including fruit mustards (see page 69), are good with mild meats, such as chicken and pork. Any of these mustards would make a wonderful addition to vinaigrettes and dressings meant for fruit salads.

Honey Mustard

This basic mild, sweet mustard has a bit of a bite that's mellowed and smoothed with a dollop of sweet honey. It's a good starter for the timid.

Spiced Honey Mustard

There are several spiced honey mustards on the market. The spices most often used are cloves and cinnamon. These mustards are particularly good with ham.

Brown Sugar and Pecan Mustard

This mustard has more than a hint of brown sugar enhanced with mellow pecans. It is almost good enough to eat over ice cream. It's excellent with cold ham.

Prickly Pear Honey Mustard

This mustard is a favorite from the deserts of the Southwest. The prickly pear comes from any cactus of the genus *Opuntia*. The fruit is shaped like a flat pear and has long thorns scattered all over it. It has soft, red flesh that is slightly sweet. This unusual mustard combines the sweetness of honey with the smoothness of the prickly pear. The result is a mild and mellow mustard. Enjoy its distinctive flavor with mild meats or in a dressing for mixed baby greens or fruit salad.

Maple Mustard

The sweetness of the maple comes through in this distinctive mild-mannered smooth mustard. This is another one that is especially good with ham.

Sesame Ginger Mustard

Sesame, ginger, and mustard are all well-known favorite flavors in Asian cooking. This mustard is a good choice as a base for a dressing for a Chinese chicken salad, and a dollop can add sweet pungency to a stir-fry.

Sweet and Hot Mustard

There are several varieties of sweet and hot mustards at your local grocery store. The sweetness usually comes from honey or corn syrup. The heat is provided by the mustard itself, but these mustards may be enhanced with peppery chilies as well. The name says it all.

FRUIT MUSTARDS

These specialty mustards have more than a hint of the distinctive sweetness of the fruits with which they are blended. Just pick your favorite fruity flavor. Fruit mustards are excellent with mild meats, and they make a good base for light and fruity vinaigrettes and the perfect glaze for chicken or duck.

Apple Mustard

This condiment contains the sweet tang of apple with the slight bite of mild mustard. It is a winner with chicken and is an excellent addition to a dressing for chicken salad.

Apricot-Ginger Mustard

Sweet and tangy apricot blended with spicy ginger and mild mustard brings a hint of the Orient to dressings of all kinds. This mustard is especially good with hot or cold pork.

Berry Mustard

Berry mustards, such as those flecked with blueberry, blackberry, or raspberry, add special fruity flavor to mild, mellow mustard. These specialty mustards bring zing to vinaigrettes. Berry mustards are good with all mild meats, including chicken and pork.

Cranberry Mustard

I am putting this ruby-red mustard in a class by itself. The tang of cranberries mated with smooth and pungent mustard makes it a favorite with many meats. At my house, it is always offered with the Thanksgiving turkey. It is equally good slathered on turkey sandwiches the next day.

Lemon Mustard

This yummy condiment contains true lemon flavor combined with the pungency of mustard. It makes an excellent addition to any sauce meant for fish, cold shrimp, or crab.

Orange and Honey Mustard

This mustard is reminiscent of sweet orange marmalade mated with mellow mustard. It is especially good with mild meats, such as chicken and pork, and makes the perfect glaze for duck. It makes a good base for fruit salad dressing, too.

Pineapple and Honey Mustard

This mustard is tart and tangy and sweet and pungent with a hint of heat. It makes a nice addition to anything Asian, including sweet and sour sauces. Try it as a glaze for skinless chicken breasts.

MUSTARDS WITH HERBS

These delectable mustards are richly flecked with herbs. You'll find many herbaceous mustards. What follows is a description of just a few. Pick your favorite and enjoy. Any light herbal mustard is especially good on a sandwich. Think of herbal mustard when preparing a sauce, too, whether for vegetables, meats, or fish.

Basil Mustard

Transform an ordinary tomato into an Italian delight with a bit of basil mustard. It's also good with cheeses and cold meats of all kinds. Try putting some basil mustard out when you're serving antipasto.

Tomato-Basil Mustard

You can't do authentic Italian anything without tomato and basil. This richly flavored mustard makes a welcome addition to the buffet table, especially when antipasto is on the menu.

Dill Mustard

When saucing any fish, think of dill mustard as a primary ingredient. This very versatile mustard is also good on a sandwich and adds real zip to roasted vegetables.

Lemon-Dill Mustard

Both lemon and dill are renowned for their way with fish. A dab of this delicious mustard can easily take the place of tartar sauce. Even if you think a mayonnaise-based tartar sauce is the only way to go, this mustard may change your mind.

Fennel Mustard

Fennel has been used for centuries as both food and medicine. Used in mustard, it adds the slightest hint of licorice flavor, with very pleasing results, indeed. It makes an interesting accompaniment to lamb.

Garlic Mustard

This one combines two of my favorite flavors in one little jar. This is an assertive mustard with pronounced garlic flavor. Garlic lovers will find it wonderful on everything from roasted vegetables to sausages to cold meats.

Garlic-Parsley Mustard

This is an interesting offering that combines the richness of garlic and the sharp cleanness of parsley with the pungency of mustard. It is especially good with cheeses and roasted vegetables.

Roasted Garlic Mustard

Roasting garlic tames this assertive herb. It smoothes out all the roughness and brings a nice mellowness while preserving the flavor. This mustard has smooth garlic flavor and mustard's pungency without being overpowering. If you like garlic, this subdued mustard is an excellent choice for sandwiches, roasted vegetables, and cold meats.

Four-Peppercorn Mustard

This grainy mustard combines the sharpness and bite of pepper with the heat and pungency of mustard. This powerhouse can hold its own when paired with hearty meats and sausages.

Rosemary Mustard

According to tradition, rosemary is for remembrance. Remember this light and flavorful mustard as a base for a dipping sauce for raw or roasted vegetables and as an addition to chicken dishes.

Rosemary-Mint Mustard

The hint of mint in this interesting mustard makes it a natural with lamb.

Tarragon Mustard

Tarragon adds its own earthy herbal signature to mustard's smooth pungency. This mustard is excellent with chicken, fish, and eggs. Try a dab the next time you make an egg salad sandwich.

HOT MUSTARDS

These hot mustards are not for the faint of heart. If you like "hot stuff," these mustards are for you. When selected ingredients are combined with mustard's fire, as in these spectacular blends, you can expect varying degrees of heat. For example, chili peppers range from mild to incindiary. Read the labels, and choose the degree of heat you want. Any of these assertive mustards can tame the spiciest meats. For more hot mustards, see Russian mustard (page 73) and German mustards (page 74).

Chipotle Pepper Mustard

Chipotle peppers from Mexico are both smoky and full of fire. Mated with mustard's heat, the result is a medium-hot mustard with heat that lingers. This mustard is good on a sandwich. A small spoonful will bring zing to any dish.

Habañero Pepper Mustard

Beware! Habañero peppers are reputed to be the hottest of the hot. When mated with the heat and fire of mustard, I am told that this inspired combination could blister paint. Try this mustard at your peril.

Horseradish Mustard

There's nothing better with rare roast beef than horseradish, and the heat of mustard just makes it even better. This mustard is excellent with all hearty meats and is a good choice with roasted vegetables, too.

Jalapeño Mustard

As peppers go, jalapeños are relatively mild. Jalapeño peppers are a staple of Tex-Mex fare. If you like that spicy cuisine, this mustard may be a favorite. A dollop served alongside the spicy Mexican sausage *chorizo* would be welcomed.

OLD WORLD MUSTARDS

With a few exceptions, most imported mustards tend to be coarse, grainy, and hearty. Some are mild, some are assertive, but any of the following mustards will complement hearty meats, including spicy kielbasa and Polish and German sausages. These mustards are wonderful with roast beef and cheeses, too.

Dutch Mustard

The *moutardes* of Holland are typically dark and flecked with specks of seeds and with a rich selection of secret spices. Mild-mannered and delicious, Dutch mustards complement the flavors of meats, cheeses, and sausages without dominating.

French Dijon Mustard

Dijon mustards imported from France are velvety smooth, heavy, and creamy in texture. Unlike with American Dijons, the French make Dijon mustard with vinegar, not wine. French Dijon mustards have true mustard flavor and are delightfully pungent, but the bite won't burn your tongue, and there's not a lot of lingering heat. Dijon mustards are excellent all-purpose mustards and are a good choice with roasted vegetables and a great dunk for pretzels.

Polish Mustard

The best Polish-style mustard I know of isn't an import—"Uncle Phil" makes it in Wisconsin. Polish mustard is dark and flecked with secret spices and is richly flavored with just the right amount of horseradish. Polish mustard is nicely pungent but not overpowering. It is perfect with sausages and cheese.

Russian Mustard

Russians like their mustard extra hot and on the sweet side. I've been told that typical Russian-style mustards bite back, so don't say you weren't warned. Russian mustards can hold their own with the spiciest meats.

Tewkesbury Horseradish Mustard

Tewkesbury mustards are so famous that Shakespeare even wrote about them. This smooth, pale mustard consists of finely powdered English mustard mated with freshly ground horseradish root, wine vinegar, and salt. Expect heat, pungency, and tang with a pleasant lingering warmth. This mustard is excellent with hot or cold roast beef and is good with roasted vegetables, too.

Swedish Mustard

Skansk senap is a heavy, creamy mustard richly flecked with spices and bits of mustard seed. This mustard is not very hot, but it is nicely pungent. It is especially good with cheese.

Sweet Austrian, Bavarian, and German Mustards

Germanic *senfs* are either very sweet or very hot. A typical German mustard is very grainy, darkly colored with secret spices, and heavily sugared. If you like sweet American-made honey mustard, a sweet German mustard is an excellent choice. These mustards are especially good with ham.

Hot Austrian, Bavarian, and German Mustards

The classic hot Germanic mustard is typically made with both brown and white mustard seeds, cold water, spirit vinegar, salt, and secret spices. It is smooth, not grainy, and a rich dark-gold color. These mustards are very hot with a definite afterburn. If you like it hot, these assertive mustards are the perfect choice to serve with the heartiest, most heavily spiced meats.

MUSTARDS WITH SPIRITS

These mustards are enriched with various alcoholic spirits. The alcohol content has vanished, but the flavor of the spirit comes through. Some of these mustards are hearty, some are delicate, but all are delicious. Guide your selection according to your liking of the taste of the various spirits.

Arran Mustard With Highland Malt Scotch

This mustard is a favorite from the Arran Isles of Scotland. Three kinds of whole mustard seeds, mellow single-malt Scotch, a hint of leek, wine vinegar, and sea salt result in a spectacular mild mustard. The jar is crowded with crunchy mustard seeds. This mustard is excellent served as a relish with all kinds of meats—hot or cold. It is perfect for sandwiches too.

Brandied Peach Mustard

This elegant and luxurious mustard is good enough to eat with a spoon. It makes a winning combination. The richness of peaches mellowed with brandy combined with the smooth pungency of mustard is delectable with chicken and pork. This mustard is excellent as a base for fruit salad, too.

Cognac Mustard

This is a hot and heavy mustard that marries the marvelous afterglow of good brandy with the heat and pungency of mustard. It is very full-flavored and smooth in the mouth. This mustard is elegant with meats and superb with roasted vegetables.

Irish "Pub" Mustard

A typical Tipperary Pub mustard is richly flavored with a brilliant combination of beer, apple juice, vinegar, secret herbs and spices, and just a touch of sugar. This grainy mustard is thick with both whole and cracked seeds. It is mild-mannered, yet packed full of flavor. It is a wonderful choice with meat or cheese.

Jack Daniel's Mustard

The black label tells you that this mustard is not just an ordinary spirited mustard. Exceedingly smooth and marvelously mellow Jack Daniel's whiskey flavors premium mustard. If you are into status symbols, this one is a must for the prestigious buffet table.

Stout Mustard

This is a smooth and pungent mustard tempered with the mellowness and warmth of a dark ale. It is medium-brown in color. This mustard is tangy and full of flavor, but warm rather than hot. It is fine for sandwiches, but is delicious with cheese and extra good for dunking pretzels.

MISCELLANEOUS MUSTARDS

Then there are those mustards that defy classification, but are so delicious, they need to be discussed somewhere. I will describe a few of those for you here.

Balsamic Mustard

Balsamic mustard, of course, is mustard mixed with smooth and mellow balsamic vinegar. It makes a rich and delicious combination. It is excellent with cold meats.

Black Olive Mustard

This mustard mates the richness of black olives and pungent mustard. The result is smooth and tangy flavor with a bit of a bite. If you're making a dip for raw vegetables, this mustard adds mellow richness.

Sun-Dried Tomato Mustard

This luscious mustard richly endowed with sun-dried-tomato flavor will enhance any sandwich. It's also another good one to keep in mind to add flavor to sauces for raw or roasted vegetables.

Maui Onion Mustard

The Maui onions of Hawaii are renowned for their sweetness. When mated with mustard, the result is a smooth and mild delight with just a bit of bite and a very pleasant aftertaste.

LET'S PARTY!

Here's an idea. The next time you decide to have a few people over, set up a mustard-tasting buffet and invite everyone to sample a variety of mustards. Provide ten or twelve mustards ranging from the classics to the exotics. If you don't know which mustards to choose, just check those I described for you for inspiration. When you set up the buffet, leave the mustards in their jars so your guests can peruse the labels.

Do provide some nibbles to dunk in the mustards. The buffet table might include slices or squares of cheese and ham, thin slices of roast beef, and any other deli delights you favor. If you decide on sliced meats and cheeses, roll them up and secure them with a toothpick. Those of you who are counting fat grams and are concerned about cholesterol should use low-fat cheese and thin-sliced turkey ham and forget the red meats.

Getting the Mustard
Out of Your Clothes

Everyone knows mustard stains are among the hardest stains to get out of clothes. Too many people have given up on a favorite blouse or pair of pants because they were stained with mustard. Well, stop throwing your clothes away! Here are some tips for getting mustard stains out of your clothes. Wipe or scrape off as much of the mustard as possible, as soon as possible. Then soak the stain in diluted bleach if the fabric is bleachable. If the fabric is not bleachable, try treating the stain with vinegar or peroxide.

Be sure to put out some cauliflower and broccoli florets, cooked just until tender-crisp and then chilled. Both these vegetables are excellent with mustard, and the dieters among your guests will gravitate to them. Everyone will welcome fresh fruit on the buffet. Some of the fruit-based mustards are marvelous with fresh fruit, especially apple and orange segments. Your guests may find fruit and mustard a surprising combination, but this pairing will meet with general approval.

Of course, everyone knows that pretzels are a natural for dunking in mustard. Select pretzel sticks, or go for the big, soft, chewy kind you can pull apart. Chunks of French bread and water biscuits are also good choices for those who want something a bit more substantial. Many breads and crackers have too much flavor of their own to let the flavor of the mustard shine through, but French bread and water biscuits are bland enough not to interfere with the taste of the various mustards.

Good beverage choices include ice-cold tomato juice, sparkling water, or a light white wine. Stay away from colas, if you can. They are so strong in taste that the palate can be dulled, and the mustards won't receive the appreciation that is their due. If you want to fuss, a simple champagne punch makes a statement that no one can ignore.

To turn your mustard-tasting into an easy buffet supper, set out a pot of bubbling fondue (see page 180 for a recipe), a platter of bread chunks, and a heaping bowlful of mixed greens lightly dressed with a mustard vinaigrette (see page 132). Let everyone help themselves at their own pace while you relax. This is one party a host and hostess can really enjoy. Once the food preparation and table setup is completed, there's nothing for the party-giver to do but join in the fun.

When I was checking supermarkets and gourmet shops and combing through catalogs in order to give you a comprehensive look at the many mustards on the market, even I was surprised to find how very many varieties of mustard are available. I kept putting jar after jar into my market basket, and I placed a large catalog order. For someone who has cooked with mustard for a long time, I confess it was an awesome experience. I was like a kid in a candy store. "Ohhh, this one will be perfect with . . ." "That one will really heat up . . ." "I must have this for . . ." And so on. I even sent some mouth-watering mustards as gifts to family members and friends who share my passion for the stuff.

Nonetheless, I want to emphasize that you don't have to have a vast selection of mustards at your disposal to make some exceptionally memorable meals. For the most part, whatever mustard you have in your refrigerator at this moment will spice up almost any dish and add zest to your table.

In the next chapter, you will learn everything you need to know to grow succulent mustard greens for your table, as well as how to harvest and dry the seeds so that you can make your own mustard.

7

Cultivating Mustard

"The mustard grows throughout Europe, except in the northeastern parts, also in South Siberia, Asia Minor, and Northern Africa, and is naturalized in North and South America. It is largely cultivated in England, Holland, Italy, Germany and elsewhere for the sake of the seed, used partly as a condiment, and partly for its oil."

—A Modern Herbal
Mrs. M. Grieve (1931)

Mustard plants have provided pungent flavor to condiments, spicy greens for the table, and medicinal compounds since time immemorial. But you do not have to buy prepared mustards or mustard greens every time you want to complement a meal with them. It is easy to grow your own mustard plants at home. Then you can harvest the seeds and prepare your own mustard, and grow your own greens for your use at any time. Mustard plants are also considered excellent feed for livestock, particularly for sheep. Mustards meant for feed can be sown just about any time. They mature so quickly, they are ready for the sheep to nibble about eight or nine weeks after being planted. White mustard is the first choice for fodder because it is less pungent than black mustard and just as nutritious. Mustard also excels as "green manure." When the plants have attained a good size, about two months after sowing, they can be plowed under, adding needed nitrogen and other nutrients to the soil.

MUSTARD'S CULTIVATION AROUND THE WORLD

Although *Brassica nigra*, black mustard, is indigenous to southern Europe, the Middle East, and Asia, it has been cultivated throughout most of Europe for centuries. It has the most pungency, the most fire, and the most flavor, which once made it a favorite of mustard producers. However, it needs a rich soil to thrive and is the most difficult to harvest. The seed pods of black mustard are brittle and must be harvested by hand, otherwise the tiny seeds can be expelled early. Today, *Brassica nigra* is grown almost exclusively in areas where the wages paid to pickers who do the laborious job of harvesting the stalks carrying seed pods by hand are shockingly low. Most black mustard is grown in Ethopia, India, and Sicily.

Because *Brassica juncea*, brown mustard, lends itself to harvesting by giant machines, it is more popular with commercial growers than the fuller-flavored black variety. In fact, brown mustard has taken the place of black mustard in many areas of the world. Its seeds are larger than those of the black variety, although they are less pungent. Brown mustard has been growing wild in China, India, Africa, and Pakistan for centuries and these countries are centers for commercial production today.

White mustard, *Sinapis alba*, is native to the Mediterranean countries and central Europe. It is now cultivated in most temperate climates around the world, including Great Britain, the United States, and Canada. In fact, Canada is one of the largest producers of white mustard seed. Since World War II, Canada has become the largest exporter of white mustard seed in the world. *Sinapis alba* grows best in heavy or sandy loam, and its seeds are the largest of the three varieties, although they are the mildest in terms of flavor and heat.

CULTIVATING MUSTARD IN YOUR GARDEN

The members of the mustard family are pretty plants. The flowers add a splash of sunny yellow to any garden. Mustard plants are annuals, meaning that they must be replanted each year in order to harvest a crop. As long as the soil is well prepared, mustard plants are not difficult to grow, and the rewards are threefold: Tender young leaves add peppery flavor to salads or pungency to the cooking pot, mustard greens are a flavorful side dish that can pep up any meal, and the seeds of all varieties are easy to harvest and easy to store. Because the seeds are so tiny, it takes a lot of mustard plants to produce a significant amount of seed. Generally speaking, you'll need at least a dozen healthy plants to yield enough seeds to make two or three batches of your own homemade mustard.

If you're going to grow your own mustard, let me suggest that you cultivate several different varieties. You can mix or match as you choose, but each member of the family has its own special traits. For example, several hybrids have been especially developed to provide tasty and tender greens.

In this chapter you'll find general guidelines to selecting and successfully growing your own mustard. In addition to following my guidelines, you should pay close attention to the instructions on the individual seed packets for the various varieties of mustard.

Selecting Your Seeds

Many home gardeners take great pleasure in leafing through seed catalogs. Catalogs are a good place to start for purchasing the right seeds, especially if you don't know exactly which mustards will suit your needs best. You'll find descriptions of the different varieties and the growing conditions they require. Some varieties mature earlier than others, which might be a factor you will need to consider, and some mustards need more specialized care than others. In areas with a temperate climate, mustard is usually planted between February and early April. Both seed packets and catalogs will tell you the best time to plant in your area of the country.

White mustard (*Sinapis alba*) is the species whose seed is most commonly used in American prepared mustards. This plant is an erect annual that grows about eighteen inches high, and the young plants are often harvested for use in salad. White mustard has a light and airy appearance, and puts forth yellow flowers. The seedpod of white mustard is hairy, roundish, and almost flat. The pod has a sword-shaped beak at its tip. The seeds of white mustard aren't really white, but yellow. Their flavor is pungent, yet mild. These seeds are somewhat larger than those of black and brown mustards.

Black mustard plants (*Brassica nigra*) are not only prolific seed producers, they are the most pungent and flavorful members of the mustard family. These plants are taller than white mustard plants. Under ideal conditions, black mustard plants can reach a height of three feet. The black mustard plant is bushier than the more delicate white mustard. Its seedpods are smooth and flattened, and its seeds are only about half the size of white mustard. If you like strong, flavorful mustard with lots of heat, black mustard is for you.

Brown mustard (*B. juncea*) is easily cultivated and has just about replaced black mustard as a commercial crop. The seeds are similar in size and color to black mustard, but the flavor is much milder. If you want mustard greens for the table, this is another good choice. The flavor of the greens of brown mustard plants is lively and peppery, and they are very nutritious. The young leaves of the brown mustard plant are highly regarded in Asia.

You can also select from several varieties of mustard that have been developed to insure a good crop of greens. For "southern-style" greens, try a variety called Green Wave. This is a large plant with curly, deeply frilled, and finely cut leaves that have a spicy flavor. Florida Broadleaf is a spreading leafy plant with oval medium-green leaves and creamy midribs. This is a hearty plant and, when boiled, the leaves make a substantial side dish for any meal. Savanna matures earlier than the other two, and offers the advantage of multiple harvests—spring and fall. The leaves are smooth, thick, dark green, and tender, but with a true mustard pungency. Southern Giant Curled is another good mustard for the gardener who likes greens. The leaves are tender, deeply cut, and frilled on the edges. This one is considered a cool season crop and should be planted in the early spring or late summer.

Most mustards can tolerate a light frost. In fact, the experts say that mustards that have been subjected to frost actually lose some of their characteristic bitterness, leaving the greens just a bit sweeter. Mustard greens develop a stronger flavor as the summer wears on. All seed packets provide a timetable showing how long it will take from planting to maturity. If you prefer milder greens, take that timetable into consideration when planting your seeds.

Preparing the Ground

In the wild, mustard makes do with whatever conditions it finds itself in. Because it is self-sowing, wild mustard often appears more prolific than it really is. Unlike with cultivated mustard, which is an annual, an overgrown mustard patch in the meadow will contain plants of various ages in various stages of growth. In many areas, mustard is considered nothing more than a troublesome weed. If mustard is allowed to "go to seed" in the garden, it will self-sow and take over the plot. It's no respecter of borders.

The cultivated varieties of mustard prefer a rich, moist, well-prepared soil with adequate drainage. The soil should be well worked at least six inches deep and should have a lot of organic matter worked in. Cultivated mustard is a hungry plant that must be well fed. If you have a compost heap, heap it on and work it in. If you do not, purchase a good organic fertilizer. For best results, the soil should have a pH of no less than 6.0. Unless you know the composition of your soil, allow one of the experts at your local nursery to guide you in choosing the best organic fertilizer for your region.

Sowing the Seed

Mustard seeds should be sown about one-quarter inch deep. You can sow the seeds directly into the plot, or start them indoors. The seeds of some varieties can be sown as close together as two inches once outdoors, while others prefer more room. The rows can be anywhere from two inches to two feet apart, depending on the variety. Follow the directions on the seed packet. It will save time later. Keep the soil of the planting bed moist, but do not soak the area. Mustards do appreciate a layer of mulch, which will keep their roots cool. Generally, you can expect the first pale green sprouts to show within one to two weeks.

When the mustard seeds are well sprouted and about one inch tall, you must thin the seedlings to make them six to eight inches apart to allow the plants enough room to mature without crowding. Do this by removing all of the seedlings every six to eight inches. In order to avoid disturbing the tiny roots of the seedlings you're planning on saving, pinch the discards off at the soil surface instead of pulling them out. Toss the tiny tender leaves of the thinnings into a salad. I know my garden is clean and pest-free, so I often eat the discards as I snick them off. The thinings are very mild and tender, with just a hint of the bite to come.

If you want to start the seeds indoors, give them four to six weeks indoors before transplanting them into their permanent home outside. To start your seeds indoors, use ordinary potting soil in flats or small peat pots. Follow the directions on the seed packet for information on how many seeds to use in a given amount of space. I favor the biodegradable peat pots. With these, the seedlings can then be planted, pots and all, in the ground, so there is less danger of disturbing the tiny roots.

For successful indoor starts, light is critical. A sunny windowsill isn't enough, nor is regular incandescent light. Fluorescent light works very well. The best lighting conditions are achieved with a double-tube setup with one cool-white fluorescent bulb and one warm-white fluorescent bulb. The tubes should be no more than three inches away from the seedlings. Give the seedlings sixteen hours of light, but no more. The idea is to create an ideal environment, while still observing the ways of nature. The seedlings need a period of dark indoors, just as they would receive outdoors.

Household temperatures of 70°F to 80°F degrees are ideal for germination, but anywhere from 60°F to 70°F degrees will work just fine. If you can manage it, give your plants a temperature drop of 10 degrees at night, just as they would receive outdoors. Think about it. A nighttime temperature drop is also part of Mother Nature's plan.

After your seedlings have been growing for about four or five weeks, it's time to begin what's known as the "hardening-off" period. You need to get your pampered plants ready for the outside world. To do that, begin acclimating the sturdy seedlings by putting them outdoors for a few hours everyday. They still need some protection, of course. Needless to say, they should stay indoors during high winds or pelting rain, just as you do when you have a choice. When the weather permits, gradually extend the time the plants spend outdoors every day. In one to two weeks, they'll be well acclimated to their new environment, and you can transplant them into their permanent location.

While starting your plants indoors will yield the best results, if all this seems like much too much trouble, be assured that you can sow mustard directly into a prepared bed outdoors and expect excellent results.

Mustard plants take the greater part of the season to produce seeds, and they appreciate a sunny summer. Be sure to follow the guidelines on the seed packet for the ideal planting conditions and season for your particular seeds. Some gardeners prefer to sow mustard seed late in the season so that the seeds will remain in the ground over the winter and yield an early crop the following season. Another advantage is that mustard sown late will produce seeds by around May of the following year. Mustards grown for greens mature sooner than seed mustards, making it possible to sow a second or even third crop between the rows in the same bed. The seed packet will indicate whether the seeds are more ideal for producing greens or seeds. If you plan on sowing additional crops throughout the season, just be sure to space your rows far enough apart to accommodate a second and third sowing.

All crops in the cabbage family, including mustard, should be rotated. Crop rotation involves planting one crop in the soil one season and then planting another crop in that soil the following season. You may then plant the first crop again the season after that. This prevents one particular plant from depleting the soil of particular nutrients. Remember, mustard is a hungry plant that rapidly depletes the soil of nutrients. That's why you shouldn't grow any member of the cabbage family in the same bed more than once every three years.

Harvesting the Plant

When you choose to harvest your mustard plants will depend upon whether you are growing the plants for their greens or for their seeds. If you're growing one of the varieties of mustard developed for greens for a salad, pick the leaves when they are young, small, and tender. For cooked greens or other uses, you will need to pick mature leaves. The leaves are mature and ready for picking when they are dark green and ten to twelve inches long. Most have a thick rib down the middle. If you're planning on adding mustard greens to a salad, select the smaller leaves. Young leaves are pungent and spicy, but not bitter. For a "mess of greens," harvest a great quantity of the large leaves from the mature plants. See Part Two for directions for cooking mustard greens.

If you want to harvest the seeds of your mustard plant so you can make your own mustard (see Part Two for directions), do this just after the seedpods take on a brownish tinge. If you allow the pods to ripen fully on the plant, they will burst open and scatter their seeds all over the ground, and you'll lose your crop. You might not think your mustard plants are producing seeds, but they are. The slender green seed vessel is hidden by the petals of the flower until the petals drop. Once the petals fall, the seed case grows into a long, lean pod with the seeds tucked inside. There may be many pods on a single stem. Each seedpod of white mustard contains from four to six globular seeds about one-twelfth of an inch in diameter. The seeds will be yellow both on the surface and in the interior. Black and brown mustard seeds are about half the size of white mustard, and each pod will yield from ten to twelve dark brown-black seeds.

The easiest way to collect the seeds is to pull the whole plant from the ground, place it in a brown paper bag, and hang it upside down in a dry place. The seeds must dry before harvesting. The time it will take for the pods to dry is affected by many variables, including air temperature and humidity and how ripe the pods were when you pulled the plant. Under optimum conditions, the seedpods should be thoroughly dry in about two weeks. Sometimes all it takes to persuade the pods to release the seeds is a good shake. In theory, the seeds will obligingly fall into the bag and you can just throw away the dried stalk with the pods still attached. It isn't usually that easy, however. You may have to break the pods open by hand and pop out the seeds. Wait at least two weeks first before trying this method.

If you're in a great hurry, break off the pods and place them in a single layer on a cookie sheet, and let them rest undisturbed until the pods are thoroughly dry. This should take about two to three days. If you have a gas stove, you can put the pods in the oven and allow the gentle heat generated by the pilot light to hasten the drying process. You may also use a dehydrator if you have one, but a microwave is not suitable for drying the seedpods.

The seedpods are dry when they no longer feel spongy to the touch. They should "crackle" when you squeeze them gently. At this point, they will open easily. Don't forget how tiny mustard seeds really are. Be sure to break the pods open over a bowl so the seeds won't roll away.

To maintain full potency, it's best to store your seeds in a glass jar with a tight lid. Although the seeds will lose some bite over time, as long as you store them properly, you can keep mustard seeds for about a year and a half without too much loss of flavor or pungency.

Incidentally, you can eat the flower buds, if you wish. In fact, if you like broccoli, you'll like mustard flower buds. Just drop them in salted boiling water for a few minutes, drain, and enjoy.

Read on to find out where you can go to learn more about mustard and how you can continue to celebrate mustard even after you finish this book.

8

A Celebration of Mustard

No matter where you travel,
No matter where you roam,
Mustard on the table
Will make you feel at home.

—Barry Levenson

I have passed on to you the most curious and amazing things I have discovered about mustard since I began writing this book. If you're still curious, you're in luck. There's more to come. For example, did you know that there are three museums that feature mustard and mustard-related items—and nothing else—in their collections? One is in England, one is in France, and one is right here in the United States. Here's a look at what you'll find if you happen to visit them.

ENGLAND'S COLMAN'S MUSTARD SHOP AND MUSEUM

It was February 15, 1823, when mustard-maker Jeremiah Colman took his nephew James into partnership and started the famous mustard-making J & J Colman firm. In 1973, the company decided to commemorate its 150th anniversary by opening Colman's Mustard Shop and Museum, the only shop of its kind in Britain. The museum features displays depicting the history of Colman's mustard from its earliest years to the present day. Old photographs, including one from 1854 showing Colman's mustard mill where mustard seed was crushed by steam-driven "stampers," are displayed, and many old and rare mustard pots are part of the museum's collection of antiques.

The shop and museum are located in picturesque Brideswell Alley in what's known as East Anglia, England. The building dates back to the 1700s, and the shop and museum have been extensively restored and decorated in late nineteenth-century style. (See Figure 8.1.) The result is a charming authentic depiction of what the museum's literature says is "a Victorian trade premises." The counters are thick marble slabs that rest atop mahogany cabinets. The rear of the shop has wooden shelves with turned posts that cover the entire wall and reach to the ceiling. The shelves display prepared mustard in pottery and metal pots, mustard powder in tins, and mustard pots and spoons. A large portrait of Queen Victoria, who is still much beloved in Britain, hangs precisely in the middle of the shelves. Even the telephone—and, yes, it works—dates back to those times. Histo-

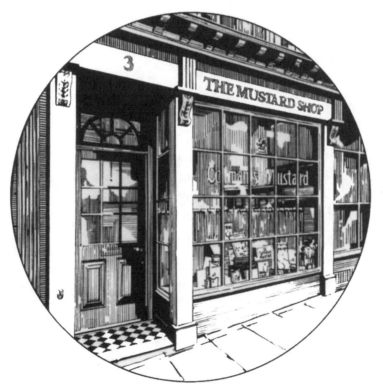

Figure 8.1. Colman's Mustard Shop & Museum, Norwich, England.

ry is very near here. It's easy to imagine a horse and carriage clopping down the narrow cobblestone street, and, look, isn't that milady's kitchen maid stopping in with a market basket over one arm?

Colman's mustard is a familiar sight in American supermarkets. I have two jars in my refrigerator right now, as well as a tin of Colman's dried mustard powder. However, Colman's Mustard Shop has more varieties of Colman's mustard than you can imagine, plus more than a dozen dried and flavored mustard powders that I have not seen in my local markets and probably never will. They also offer an extensive collection of mustard pots and spoons, including some reproductions from Colman's early days. Mugs, tea towels, and novelty items such as magnets, bookmarks, and toys are also available. Both the shop and museum are popular tourist attractions. If you're traveling to England and want to stop in, you'll find their address and phone number in the Resources section of this book. If you can't get there, but want to try a true taste of old England, Colman's Mustard Shop also sells by mail and will be happy to send you a catalog.

FRANCE'S MOUTARDE MAILLE SHOPS AND MUSEUM

The first gourmet shop in France was opened in 1747 by Master Antoine Maille on the Rue Saint-Andre des Arts in Paris. One of his contemporaries said of Maille, "From an industry, an art was made." This premiere mustard-maker was so renowned that he was called "Master," not merely monsieur or mister. The House of Maille has been making mustard for over 250 years, and the motto of the firm remains that of the founder: excellence, diligence, and refinement. During his time, Master Maille was called the greatest mustard- and vinegar-maker of all time. Master Maille's products were so fine that he became the official mustard and vinegar supplier to the great courts of Europe.

Boutique Maille in Paris and Le Musée Amora Boutique Moutarde Maille in Dijon (see Figures 8.2 and 8.3) offer a great variety of French-style condiments, with an emphasis on mustards. If you were shopping at Maille in eighteenth-century Paris, your mustard would have been served up from an earthenware pump and packed in a stoneware pitcher bearing the symbol of the House of Maille. Interestingly enough, customers shopping for freshly prepared Maille mustard will find it is still pumped and packaged before their very eyes in the same way today. As far as I have been

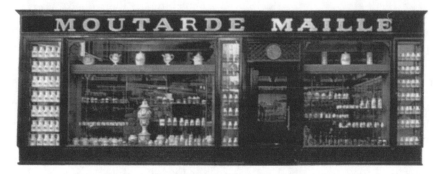

Figure 8.2. Boutique Maille, Paris, France.

able to determine, Maille's boutiques are the only shops where freshly made mustard is still sold.

The shops also offer condiments described as "of a rare richness prepared to satisfy the most classical tastes to the most daring savours." The Maille boutiques sell fifty different condiments, including a full range of original Maille mustards, all fit for the most discriminating epicure. You can also choose from a wide selection of flavored vinegars, five varieties of gherkins (prickly fruit of a West Indian vine sold as curiosities), and a whole range of pickled fruits and vegetables, including olives, onions, peppers, and capers. Unfortunately, the shops do not offer the convenience of mail-order shopping.

Moutarde Maille in Dijon, where mustard has been made for centuries, is home to Le Musée Amora. This museum contains an extensive and quite fascinating collection of old photographs related to mustard-making, as well as poster art dating back to the mid-

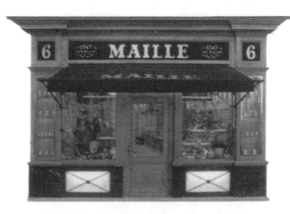

Figure 8.3. Boutique Moutarde Maille & Le Musée Amora, Dijon, France.

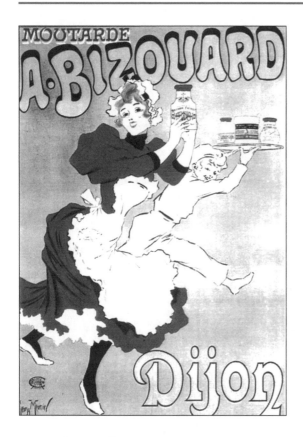

Figure 8.4. 1896 poster advertising Moutarde A. Bizouard.
Courtesy of Le Musée Amora, Dijon, France.

1800s. All of these early advertisements are very colorful. There's even one dated 1896 that is very reminiscent of Toulouse-Lautrec's distinctive style (See Figure 8.4.) Many of the mustard pots displayed in the museum are even older than the art.

In 1785, a French clipper ship carrying a shipload of Maille's potted mustard and vinegar destined for the Russian court sank off the coast of Finland. No doubt the tsar was disappointed when it didn't arrive. The submerged wreck was discovered and salvage operations were mounted in 1979. The museum has on exhibit an eighteenth-century mustard pot that was brought up from the wreck. This pot is made of fine china and is clearly identified as containing mustard made by Master Maille. (See Figure 8.5.) Note that this mustard pot has the narrow neck and flared top characteristic of mustard pots of old times. It would have been tightly sealed with a cork or thick wax plug. Because this mustard was traveling by ship, it was most likely first stoppered with a cork and then double-sealed with wax.

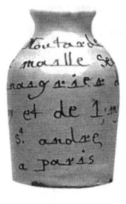

Figure 8.5. Eighteenth
century Maille mustard
pot salvaged from a ship
sunk in 1785. The cargo
was consigned to the
Russian court.
Courtesy of Le Musée
Amora, Dijon, France.

If you're interested in mustard, antique and contemporary mustard pots, and old mustard art, you'll find the addresses of Boutique Maille in Paris and Le Musée Amora Boutique Moutarde Maille in Dijon in the Resources section near the end of this book. I know you'll want to stop in the next time you're in France.

UNITED STATES' THE MOUNT HOREB MUSTARD MUSEUM

Both the English and French museums are connected to a mustard-maker, and feature only the mustard-maker's brand of mustard; however, the Mount Horeb Mustard Museum of Mount Horeb, Wisconsin, is very different. The founder and curator of this museum, Barry Levenson, has set himself to the task of collecting a sample of every mustard in the universe. This former attorney is a formidable force in the world of mustard. He wrote the foreword to this book. I love his writing style. I'm sure you will, too. In the foreword, Barry tells you in his own words how mustard became a personal obsession that eventually evolved into the only mustard museum on this continent.

In a short ten years, the museum collection has grown to an astounding 2,915 pots, jars, and boxes of different varieties of mustard from every state in the United States, and other countries are represented as well. More mustards are coming in all the time. Friends of the museum make a point of bringing Barry exotic mustards collected in their travels. The museum also has a collection of 1,300 mustard pots, including some rare Fiestaware pots (which are prized by collectors), on display. Many of the pots date back to the 1800s, and some are lined with brilliant blue cobalt glass. In case you don't remember, let me remind you that a glass lining was a feature of early mustard pots. It was needed to prevent the acid content of mustard from eating into the metal pots.

By 1991, Barry's love affair with mustard was so well known that he was asked to be chairman of National Mustard Day, celebrated annually on the first Saturday in August. Before he took over, National Mustard Day was sponsored by the Plochman Mustard Company of Chicago. And, yes, National Mustard Day is a recognized holiday. You'll not only find it listed in *Chase's Calendar of Events*, the comprehensive day-by-day book that lists every holiday, event, and festival imaginable, but it's been read into the Congressional Record as a holiday.

Barry is also the guiding light of the World Mustard Association (WMA), established in 1997 in conjunction with mustard-makers everywhere. Companies with a connection to mustard can become "related business associate members." Such organizations are welcome if they sell to mustard-makers, or manufacture food products that cry out for mustard, such as pretzels and hot dogs. Ordinary people with an interest in mustard can become "associate members." Membership advantages include an informative WMA pamphlet and discounts on special items available for sale at the museum.

In addition, Barry created "Poupon U," a mythical university dedicated to mustard education. My doctorate in mustard from Poupon U testifies that I have successfully completed my mustard studies and am an authentic Doctor of Mustard. (See Figure 8.6 on page 94.) If you attend a pep rally, I want you to be prepared. Here's the school's cheer:

> *Who needs Harvard, who needs Yale?*
> *At Poupon U, you'll never fail!*
> *Stanford, Princeton? Big mistake!*
> *Poupon U's a piece of cake.*

If you want your doctorate, you'll have to take the final exam. It's in the museum literature, but don't worry, you can't fail. The answers are included with the exam, and Barry says it's OK to peek before turning in your paper.

One of the most interesting things Barry is involved in is the Mustard Family Reunion. As the museum became increasingly well-known, people with the surname Mustard began calling. Soon there were so many Mustards on the client list that a family reunion

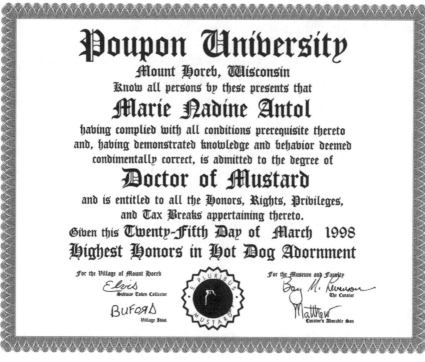

Figure 8.6. Doctorate in Mustard Diploma.

seemed inevitable. In order to reach all the Mustards possible, Barry used a CD/ROM program to find Mustard families, and sent out a mailing announcing the First Mustard Family Reunion. That reunion occurred in July of 1997, and close to 100 families attended. It was so successful that it has become an annual event.

Although I don't believe he attended the Mustard Family Reunion, perhaps the most well-known Mustard of all is "Colonel Mustard," made famous by the board game Clue. I wanted to find out just how Colonel Mustard came into being. Carrying all of this one step beyond ridiculous, I was delighted to find a history of sorts on this charmer in the novelty clothing catalog, the *J. Peterman* Winter 1997 catalog. There, I found the following story on what they call "the man behind the myth." According to the catalog, Colonel Mustard was born in 1885 and followed family tradition by going into the military. He served with distinction and was awarded the Military Cross in the Great War as a Major in the Second Battalion of the Royal Welsh Fusiliers (a segment of the British Army). Mustard was subsequently promoted to colonel and served in India with First Earl

Mountbatten of Burma, the British naval officer who was the last viceroy and governor-general of India. After his distinguished military career, he retired to Kings Nympton in Devon, England. The catalog copy continues by saying that the Colonel likes a sharp crease and has a predilection for herringbone trousers. If you ever talk with the Colonel, the catalog has a bit of advice: "Speak loudly; he's 114."

You might also want to check out Barry Levenson's "Colonel Mustard: The True Story," published in *The Wurst of the Proper Mustard*, which includes the above story, as well as selections from the newsletters from 1988 to 1993 published by the "incurable curator" of the museum. This twenty-four-page delight is available for a small price through the museum.

The Mount Horeb Mustard Museum catalog offers a fascinating look at more types of mustards than you ever knew existed, all available by mail order. You can also purchase pennants, tee shirts, and sweatshirts emblazoned with the Poupon U logo. And this catalog offers mustard pots, mustard mugs, and even mustard baths and mustard rubs. If it is in any way related to mustard, you'll find it in the museum catalog. This is the best source I know of for everything related to mustard, and the twice-yearly newsletter Barry puts out for his clients is both informative and amusing. The address and 800 number for the museum are in the Resources section of this book. By the way, if you're planning to visit the museum, you won't get lost on the way. Mount Horeb is the only city I know of that lists "mustard" (along with gas, food, and lodging) on the sign that points the way into town. (See Figure 8.7.)

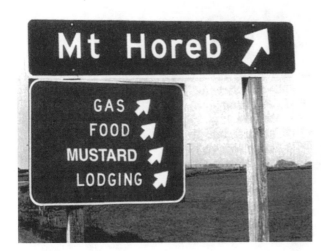

Figure 8.7.
Highway sign pointing the way to Mt. Horeb's many attractions.

THE NAPA VALLEY MUSTARD FESTIVAL

California's Napa Valley is famous around the world as the heart of wine country, so thoughts of this region inevitably bring wine to mind. Change your mindset right now and prepare to celebrate Mustard Season in Napa Valley. For two months every spring, wine takes a back seat to mustard. The Mustard Festival begins in early February, when the wild mustard blooms and carpets the valley with golden-yellow flowers that dance in the wind, and continues through the month of March. This is the time of year when the celebrated vineyards are brown and the trees are just beginning to bud. The golden flowers of the wild mustard that cover the land and follow the rolling hills as far as the eye can see are a dazzling sight.

"Madame Mustard," an original painting by Jessel Miller, was the official poster of the 1998 Mustard Festival. (See Figure 8.8.) It's a beautiful melange of regal colors, including golds and purples and reds and greens, all muted, but infused with the soft light of Napa Valley sunshine. I don't know how they will top this effort in future years. Jessel has also written a charming children's book entitled *Mustard—A Story About Soft Love and Strong Values*, which has been very well received. Her book features twenty-four original paintings done in the same inimitable Jessel style. The paintings were exhibit-

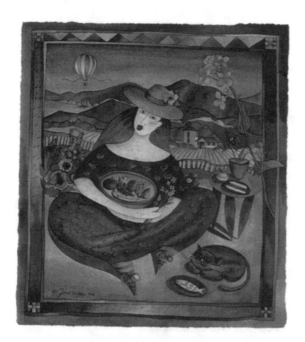

Figure 8.8. Madame Mustard, by Jessel Miller.

Official poster of the 1998 Napa Valley Mustard Festival.

ed and the book was released to great applause during the Mustard Magic event that opened the festival.

The Worldwide Mustard Competition is another feature of the festival that draws mustard makers from around the world who bring their wares to be judged. As you might imagine, the competition is fierce. The winners in the different categories immediately trumpet the news on their labels and in their advertising, and why not? Winning this prestigious event is a real feat. Shoppers take delight in the Mustard Marketplace, which features mustards from around the world, gourmet foods, Napa Valley cuisine presented by renowned Napa Valley chefs, craft brews, cooking demonstrations, fine art, exquisite crafts for food and wine lovers, art projects for children, and historic exhibits. There's also a Mustard Recipe Competition that culminates with the crowning of The Napa Valley Chef of the Year. You'll find some exceptional prize-winning mustard recipes from the 1998 event in Part Two. Wine is featured in many events—this is wine country, after all—but mustard rules. There are benefit wine auctions, art and photography competitions, and a multitude of food, wine, and entertainment events, including mustard menus, tastings, dinners, and the Napa Valley Mustard Festival Golf Benefit.

The two-month-long Mustard Season is one of the most exciting times to visit Napa Valley. Few people have the luxury of staying for the entire two months, so it's next to impossible to give an exact count of the number of people in attendance; however, officials estimate that between 50,000 and 100,000 very happy people came and went during the 1998 festival.

If you're interested in planning a springtime visit to Napa Valley during Mustard Season, make a call to Summers McCann, the firm that plans the festival, or check out their website on the Internet. You'll find them listed in the Resources section toward the back of the book. Perhaps I'll see you there!

MUSTARD'S USE AROUND THE GLOBE

I don't believe there is any country on planet Earth where mustard is not the most important condiment on the table. It is used to spice up food worldwide. I have it on good authority that the French are Europe's largest and most enthusiastic producers of mustard, which includes the master mustard-makers of Dijon. In 1996, the last year for which figures are available, the twelve mustard-makers of

The World Traveler's Guide to Mustard

As the ditty at the beginning of this chapter states—"No matter where you come from/ No matter where you roam/ Mustard on the table/ Will make you feel at home." It would help if you could ask for mustard to put on the table no matter where you are. Here is your guide for asking for mustard in fifty-four languages.

Language	Mustard Translation
Arabic	hardal
Armenian	mananekh
Bengali	sorisa
Bomenian	horčice
Burmese	moun-nyīn
Cantonese	gaailaaht
Chinese	chieh-mo
Cornish	kedhow
Croatian	mustarda or gorusica
Czech	horčice
Danish	senep
Dutch	mosterd
Fijian	masitedi
Gaellic	sgeallan
German	mostrich or senf
Greek	mostarda
Hawaiian	mākeke
Hebrew	hardal
Hindi (Urdu)	sarso
Hokkien	gkaihluā
Hungarian	mustár
Indian	svetarsarisha
Indonesian	moster
Irish	mustaird

Language	Mustard Translation
Italian	senape or mostarda
Japanese	Karashi or masotadah
Kampuchean	gaylaat
Korean	kyŏ-ja or geja
Lao	nammâhk-pētlĕuang
Latin	sinapi
Malay	mostar
Mandarin	jiémó
Norwegian	sennep
Pali	sasapa or siddhattha
Persian (Farsi)	khārdal
Pidgin	mastet
Polish	musztarda
Portuguese	a mostarda
Rumanian	mustar
Russian	mastəd or gorchitsa
Samoan	'ava āluga
Sinhalese	aba
Spanish	mostaza
Swahili	haradali
Swedish	senap
Tagalog	mustasa
Tahitian	muta
Tamil	kadugu
Thai	nām jim hahsdtāht
Tongan	masitati
Turkish	hardal
Ukranian	mastəd or gorchitsa
Vietnamese	mu-tac or bôt hạt cái
Welsh	mwstard

—Courtesy of Barry Levenson, Curator, The Mount Horeb Mustard Museum

France produced 68,188 tons of the golden condiment. The French consume around a pound-and-a-half (0.85 kilogram) of the golden delight per year per person.

Germany has the second-highest production record, with nineteen mustard-makers producing 63,114 tons of various mustards in 1996. My German correspondent tells me that the tastes of the Germans vary. In the north, people prefer medium-hot or pungent mustards. In the southern part of the country, sweet mustards made with sugar or honey are favored. These mustards are usually called Bavarian mustard. Countrywide, each German eats around a pound-and-a-quarter (0.72 kilogram) of their favorite mustard every year.

Although the Austrians seem to like mustard with tarragon best, their production doesn't keep up with their consumption. With each Austrian consuming about two-and-a-quarter pounds (1.03 kilogram) of mustard per year, you might be surprised to learn that the people of Austria have the highest per capita consumption of mustard in Europe. In 1996, the country's eight mustard-makers produced only 8,240 tons of the golden condiment.

In England, the market for prepared mustards is small in comparison to powdered mustard. Except for the ever-popular Colman's prepared mustards, it seems the British still prefer to mix dry mustard with cold water and vinegar just before serving it. I don't have per capita consumption figures for the Brits, but I can tell you that in 1996, the four mustard-producers of the United Kingdom turned out 4,700 tons of mustard.

In Italy, 1996 production figures tallied 1,245 tons and consumption totaled about half a pound (.04 kilogram) per person. Belgium produced 2,310 tons, and per capita consumption was about a pound (.47 kilogram). Spain produced 1,376 tons, and each Spaniard ate a little under a pound (.06 kilogram) of mustard.

And that, dear reader, concludes the educational, informative, interesting, and amusing Part One. I'm sure you learned some things you didn't know about mustard, the phenomenal golden herb-spice-medicinal-condiment.

You are now invited to turn the pages and peruse Part Two, Mustard Recipes.

Part Two
Mustard Recipes

In this section of the book, you'll learn how to make your own homemade mustards with all the seeds you'll be harvesting, as well as how to personalize store-bought mustards with your own favorite ingredients. You'll also find several ways to enjoy mustard greens. If you don't want to grow your own, that's all right, too. This section contains a wealth of recipes that feature mustard, whether purchased or homemade.

INGREDIENT CONSIDERATIONS

A tablespoon of basic yellow prepared mustard contains 15 calories, and less than a tenth of a gram of fat. One tablespoonful also contains 18 milligrams of calcium, 7 milligrams of magnesium, and 21 milligrams each of phosphorus and potassium, plus traces of iron, copper, and zinc. Unless a particular mustard is specified in a recipe, use your favorite mustard in these dishes. There are many to choose from. In most cases, any mustard will add the characteristic flavor and pungency needed in these recipes. In some recipes, a specific mustard is called for; for example, honey mustard is best for Honey Mustard Salad Dressing (of course). For the rest of the recipes, experiment and use the mustard of your choice. Whatever mustard you choose, the flavor will meld deliciously with the other ingredients to result in a memorable dish. That's a promise.

Oils, Fats, and Cholesterol

Though there is much talk in the media today about reducing cholesterol in one's diet, cholesterol is essential to the body. Only about 20 percent of the cholesterol in your body is obtained in your food; the other 80 percent is produced by the liver. Cholesterol is present in the blood, the brain, liver, kidneys, adrenal glands, and the fatty "cushion" around nerve fibers. The body needs cholesterol for the manufacture of vitamin D and various hormones, including sex hormones, and it's required for the utilization of fatty acids. Nonetheless, caution is in order. Everyone knows by now that cholesterol has been implicated in the formation of the nasty plaque that can build up in the arteries, narrowing the passageways and causing heart problems. Although animal-based products—including meats, natural cheeses, whole milk, butter, and eggs—do not foster the development of free radicals, they do contain the saturated fats and cholesterol that have the potential to create health problems. The body needs a bit of fat, but too much of any kind of fat in the diet is a risk factor for many conditions of ill health. Practice moderation.

A tablespoon of any oil contains 14 grams of fat and 100 calories. If the fat is of plant origin—such as olive or canola oils—it will contain no cholesterol at all. If it is of animal origin—such as butter—1 tablespoonful will contain 30 milligrams of cholesterol. Oils such as olive and canola oil contain monounsaturated fat—the type of fat that appears to reduce levels of the LDL cholesterol—the "bad" cholesterol—in the blood. Animal-based fats and oils contain saturated fat—the blood-cholesterol raising type of fat. Certain fish oils and other plant oils, such as corn, sunflower, soybean, and safflower oils, contain polyunsaturated fat, which lowers blood levels of the bad cholesterol, but also lowers levels of HDL cholesterol—the "good" cholesterol—in the blood.

The January 1998 issue of *Archives of Internal Medicine* (published by the American Medical Association) contained a report that followed more than 60,000 subjects. This study showed that eating just 10 grams (about three-quarters of a tablespoon) of monounsaturated fats daily, found in olive and canola oils, may reduce the risk of some cancers. This study also determined that eating just 5 grams (about one-third of a tablespoon) of polyunsaturated fats daily, found in common vegetable oils, margarines, salad dressings, and many quick-fix foods, increases the formation of free radicals that can damage DNA and promote tumor development, thereby increasing the risk of some types of cancer by 69 percent. If you want to avoid these fats, and you should, read labels carefully.

A few of the recipes in the following chapters call for a tablespoon or two of butter, and one or two call for heavy cream. However, for the most part, olive oil or canola oil is specified in these recipes. By now, you've probably seen a number of articles citing the dangers of hydrogenated and partially hydrogenated fats, which contain trans-fatty acids. Trans-fatty acids have been shown to raise LDL cholesterol and lower HDL cholesterol. I've been writing about the problems these fats can cause for over ten years now. They have no place in my household, and shouldn't be in yours.

Dairy Products and Eggs

For a very long time, I have been serving my family nothing but nonfat milk. I also use nonfat sour cream exclusively, and no one complains. Where milk is called for in the following recipes, either low-fat or nonfat milk works fine. We've had more trouble switching to reduced-fat cheeses, but mustard provided the solution. I have found that the low-fat and nonfat cheese products, which are sometimes lacking in flavor, are greatly improved by the addition of mustard. Cheese and mustard go together so perfectly that I can't imagine a cheese dish without it. Don't hesitate to try the low-cal, low-fat recipes in the following chapters because you fear the resulting dish will be bland. The zip that mustard brings to the dishes makes all the difference.

One large egg contains 70 calories, 4.5 grams of fat, 215 milligrams of cholesterol, and 6 grams of protein. However, raw eggs may also contain harmful bacteria, such as *Salmonella*. In order to kill these harmful bacteria, it's necessary to cook them thoroughly. Even scrambled eggs should be cooked until dry, and eggs "over-easy" or "sunny-side-up" remain only pleasant memories. This is why the recipes that do not require cooking call for egg substitute rather than eggs. Another advantage to the use of egg substitutes is that they do not contain cholesterol. One-quarter cup of egg substitute is equivalent to one whole egg.

The recipes in the following chapters have come from many sources. Some are family recipes, and others came from friends. I am also privileged to be able to give you some recipes from the renowned Napa Valley chefs who participated in the 1998 Napa Valley Mustard Festival. Still others are adaptations of recipes I clipped at one time or another from magazines and newspapers, and some, taken from published cookbooks, have been given some special touches of my own. Bon appétit!

Mustard Creams

*The seede of Mustard pounded with vinegar is an
excellent sauce, good to be eaten with any meates, either
fish or flesh, because it doth help the digestion, warmeth
the stomache, and provoketh appetite.*

— *The Herball, or Generall Historie of Plantes*
John Gerard (1545–1612)

The mustard cream recipes that follow run the gamut from the basics to the exotics. All call for cold water. Remember, it's cold water that causes the chemical reaction that releases the heat and pungency of the seed. With the exception of a few mustards, these recipes make only a small amount of mustard, usually enough for a family meal. If you discover you really like a particular homemade mustard, feel free to double or triple the recipe. Enjoy.

For the adventurous, I have provided recipes for preparing your own mustard creams from scratch. The first step in making mustard is to crack, crush, or grind the seeds. To crack or crush the seeds, you can use a mortar and pestle or the back of a spoon, or you can whack the seeds between two layers of foil with a hammer, but it's not easy to do. One tablespoon of mustard seeds will yield one tablespoon of mustard powder. Mustard seeds are tough. The best, easiest, and most thorough way to prepare the seeds for mustard making is to grind them in a seed or coffee grinder. A blender can't "cut the mustard." If you decide to use your coffee grinder, be aware that it won't be fit for grinding coffee beans ever again. No matter how well you think you've cleaned it, you'll end up with a hint of a mustard taste in your coffee cup.

Using a seed grinder will allow you to reduce the seeds to a powder. You may sift out the hulls, if you like, or you can pulse the grinder on and off and end up with a coarser grind. I happen to like fine powder blended with coarsely ground seeds best. This combination mixes up into an earthy, grainy mustard that provides a burst of flavor in the mouth. However, if you don't have a fine harvest of seeds, or if you don't want to bother doing your own grinding, you can buy mustard powder and start with that.

Basic Yellow Mustard

This is the familiar "ballpark" type mustard that everyone
likes best on hot dogs. It's also what many delicatessens
slather on sandwiches of all types.

YIELD: 4 TABLESPOONS

3 tablespoons dry mustard powder

1 1/2 tablespoons turmeric

1 1/2 teaspoons sugar

1/4 teaspoon salt

1 teaspoon vinegar

Cold water

1. In a small bowl, mix the dry ingredients together.

2. Add the vinegar and drizzle in just enough water to form a
paste. Mix well.

No-Cook Fat-Free Mustard Cream

This cream is an excellent choice for serving as a dip with a tray
of chilled broccoli, cauliflower florets, and slivered carrots.
Dieters in the crowd will thank you.

YIELD: 1/2 CUP

1/2 cup fat-free sour cream

2 teaspoons of your favorite prepared mustard

1/4 teaspoon salt

1/8 teaspoon paprika

Mix all of the ingredients together. For full flavor, wait 30 minutes
after preparation before serving.

Non-Dairy Mustard Cream

There are those who for one reason or another avoid dairy products
in their diets. This mustard cream is great for such people.
It makes a delicious dip, and it serves equally well in
any dish where you want the tang of mustard.

YIELD: 1/2 CUP

3 tablespoons dry mustard powder

3 tablespoons water

2 tablespoons chickpea flour (available in most grocery stores)

2 teaspoons lemon juice or vinegar

2 teaspoons sugar

Mix all of the ingredients together in a small bowl to form a smooth paste. For best flavor, wait 30 minutes before serving.

Dijon-Style Mustard

True Dijon mustard is made with white wine, as called for in this
recipe. Making your own Dijon-style mustard at home is a cost-
effective way to enjoy the flavor of France at any time you like.

YIELD: 1/2 CUP

1/4 cup dry mustard powder

1/8 cup cold water

1/4 cup white wine

1/2 teaspoon salt

1/2 teaspoon sugar

1. Mix the mustard with the water in a small bowl, then add the wine to make a paste.

2. Add the sugar and salt and combine well.

Faux Fancy Mustard

In this chapter, I provide you with some recipes for making your own mustard creams; however, I am sure that there are many of you who will not want to bother making homemade mustard—although I assure you it's both easy and fun to do. For you, here are guidelines for personalizing store-bought mustard with your choice of ingredients, with just a little fuss.

Doctoring up store-bought mustard is easy to do. Just purchase a jar of basic stone-ground or whole-grain mustard that contains no extra spices, herbs, fruits, or spirits, and add the flavors of your choice. You don't even have to doctor up the whole jar all at once.

A single 8-ounce jar of mustard can easily be divided into quarters (about one-quarter cup, or 4 tablespoons, each), and each quarter can be "fancied up" with the addition of different ingredients. In my house, everyone wants something different. You know what makes a hit in your household. This is an easy and economical way to satisfy everyone.

Simply measure out 4 tablespoons of mustard, put them in a small bowl, and add the ingredients you know will please someone special or yourself. There may be someone who can't get enough garlic. Easy—blend in half a minced or roasted clove of garlic. Some like it hot, so add a teaspoon of horseradish root (either dried or preserved), or a teaspoon of crushed hot peppers, or even a drop or two of hot pepper sauce. For those who like sweet mustard, add 2 teaspoons of honey or a tablespoon of sieved orange marmalade, a personal favorite of mine. For a mellow flavor, add a teaspoon or two of spirits, such as a dark ale, beer, or whiskey. You may sometime need, say, a tarragon mustard for a particular recipe. For a fragrant herbed mustard, add a teaspoon of dried and crumbled tarragon, or any herb of your choice. After the extra ingredients are smoothly blended in, cover the bowl. To give the flavors time to meld, let the mustard steep for at least thirty minutes before serving.

I hope you will use these recipes as a jumping off point. Don't hesitate to experiment with your favorite flavors. When you become a master mustard-maker, keep in mind that homemade mustard is a welcome hostess gift. Put your homemade mustard cream creation in a pretty jar or small crock and cap it. For a "country touch," put the crock into the center of a checkered or gingham napkin, bring the four corners up, and tie several strands of raffia around the top "hobo-style." If the country look isn't suitable for the person you wish to give a gift to, perhaps you'll be lucky enough to find a pressed or cut glass jar in an antique store (or grandmother's attic) to hold your mustard cream. Top the jar with a cork or layer of paraffin. For a "formal" presentation, use an old (or new) damask napkin, and tie up the four corners with black and silver ribbon.

Spirited Mustard

This is another hearty mustard that will stand up to hearty fare.

YIELD: 2 CUPS

$\frac{1}{4}$ cup dry mustard powder

$\frac{1}{4}$ cup coarsely ground mustard seed
(If coarsely ground seed is not available, increase amount of dry mustard powder to $\frac{1}{2}$ cup instead.)

$\frac{1}{4}$ cup cold water

$\frac{1}{4}$ cup spirit of your choice, such as wine, whiskey, Scotch, ale, or beer

$\frac{1}{2}$ tablespoon light brown sugar

$\frac{1}{4}$ teaspoon salt

1. In a small saucepan, mix the cold water into the mustard powder and seeds to make a paste. Slowly add the spirits of your choice.

2. Simmer over very low heat, stirring constantly, for about fifteen minutes, or until the mixture thickens. The alcohol will boil away, but the flavor of the spirit will remain.

3. Stir in the sugar and salt and continue simmering, stirring constantly, for another 5 minutes.

4. The flavor intensifies as the sauce cools, but this mustard may be served warm, if you wish.

Elegant Mustard Cream

*Mild and pungent all at once, this true mustard
cream is a wonderful "dunk" for crudites.
It's also very good on roasted vegetables.*

YIELD: 1/2 CUP

2 tablespoons dry mustard powder

1–2 teaspoons cold water

1/2 cup heavy cream (or evaporated milk) whipped until stiff

Pinch salt (optional)

Pinch paprika (optional)

1. Mix together the mustard powder and water until the mixture is the consistency of a thin cream.

2. Fold the mustard mixture into the whipped cream or evaporated milk.

3. Add salt and paprika, if desired.

Mustard-Mayonnaise

*A Dijon mustard/mayonnaise combination has become a very
popular choice since it came on the market not long ago. By mixing
it up at home, you can make as much as you need for a few
sandwiches without buying a whole jar.*

YIELD: 6 TABLESPOONS

4 tablespoons fat-free mayonnaise

2 tablespoons prepared Dijon-Style Mustard (see page 107 for recipe)

Mix the mayonnaise and mustard together in a small bowl ten minutes before serving. The delay allows the full flavor of the mustard to permeate the mayonnaise.

Sweet Honey Mustard

Honey mustard was first popularized by delis. It's the first choice of many for ham sandwiches and barbecued meats.

YIELD: $1/2$ CUP
3 tablespoons dry mustard powder
1 $1/2$ tablespoons cold water
1 teaspoon vinegar
1 tablespoon canola oil
2 tablespoons honey

1. Mix the cold water and vinegar into the dry mustard to make a thick paste.

2. Blend in the oil and the honey, and mix until very smooth.

Sweet 'n' Easy Orange Mustard

This recipe can make your reputation as a master mustard-maker, and it's so easy. Try it for yourself.

YIELD: ABOUT $1/4$ CUP
3 tablespoons dry mustard powder
1 tablespoon cold water
1 tablespoon orange marmalade

1. Mix the dry mustard with the cold water in a small bowl to form a paste.

2. Force the orange marmalade through a sieve to break up any chunks. Add the sieved marmalade to the mustard mixture, and mix well.

3. Allow the mixture to sit for 30 minutes before serving to combine flavors.

Tangy Orange Honey Mustard

Tangy and fruity all at once, this mustard is an excellent choice as a complement to cold meats, as well as a base for a fruit salad dressing.

YIELD: 1/4 CUP

3 tablespoons dry mustard powder
1 1/2 tablespoons cold water
1 teaspoon vinegar
1 tablespoon honey
1 tablespoon orange zest*
1/2 tablespoon canola oil

*When grating an orange for zest, avoid the bitter white membrane found just under the orange peel.

1. Mix the cold water and vinegar into the dry mustard to make a thick paste.

2. Blend in the honey, orange zest, and oil. Mix until very smooth.

Hot Horseradish Mustard

This mustard is the traditional choice for serving with roast beef. Try this one on hearty sausages, such as bratwurst and kielbasa.

YIELD: 3/4 CUP

1/2 cup dry mustard powder
1/4 cup cold water
1 1/2 tablespoons horseradish root, grated or prepared
1 teaspoon brown sugar
1 teaspoon salt
1/2 cup white vinegar

1. In a small saucepan, combine the mustard and water. Stir well to make a paste.

2. In a separate bowl, combine the horseradish, sugar, and salt. Add to the mustard mixture.

3. Slowly stir in the vinegar, and combine well.

4. Simmer over very low heat, stirring constantly until the mixture thickens.

Herbaceous Mustard

No matter which herb you choose to use for this recipe, this fine mustard sauce is as delicious warm over vegetables as it is as a sandwich spread.

YIELD: 2 CUPS
¼ cup dry mustard powder
¼ cup coarsely ground mustard seed (If coarsely ground seed is not available, increase amount of dry mustard powder to ½ cup instead.)
¼ cup cold water
¼ cup dry white wine or white wine vinegar
½ tablespoon light brown sugar
¼ teaspoon salt
2 teaspoons dried tarragon, dill, basil, thyme, oregano, or rosemary (crushed)

1. In a small saucepan, mix the cold water into the mustard powder and seeds to make a paste.

2. Slowly add the white wine or white wine vinegar.

3. Simmer over very low heat, stirring constantly, for about fifteen minutes or until the mixture thickens.

4. Stir in the sugar and salt and continue simmering, stirring constantly, for another 5 minutes.

5. Remove from heat, and stir in the herb of your choice.

6. The flavor intensifies as the sauce cools, but it may be served warm, if you wish.

Danish Mustard

This mustard is sweet and sour and spicy and mellow—all at the same time. It is excellent with any meat dish.

YIELD: ABOUT 2 CUPS

⅔ cup dry mustard powder

½ cup dark brown sugar

¼ cup apple cider vinegar

1 teaspoon Worcestershire sauce

1 teaspoon lemon juice

Salt and pepper to taste

¼ cup olive oil

1. Whisk all ingredients together, adding the oil slowly. You may use a blender if you wish to insure that the ingredients don't separate upon standing.

2. This mustard needs to mellow. Place in a tightly capped jar in the refrigerator for 3 days before serving.

Chinese Mustard

This is "real" Chinese mustard as opposed to those little packets often served in fast-food Chinese restaurants. The vinegar intensifies the heat, and the oil gives it a gloss. I love it. Make only the amount you need for a meal. This is not a "keeper," as the flavor diminishes with time.

YIELD: 3 TABLESPOONS

2 tablespoons dry mustard powder

1 tablespoon cold water

1 teaspoon vinegar

½ teaspoon sesame oil

1. Combine the mustard powder and cold water. You may adjust the amount of cold water to make a thicker or thinner sauce to suit your personal preference.

2. Add the vinegar and sesame oil. Serve immediately.

Roasted Garlic Mustard

If garlic is your passion, this mustard is for you. Because the garlic is roasted, it's deliciously mellow. This mustard is good with hearty meats, such as roast beef and sausages.

YIELD: $\frac{1}{2}$ CUP
3 tablespoons dry mustard powder
1 $\frac{1}{2}$ tablespoons cold water
1 teaspoon vinegar
1 tablespoon roasted garlic, mashed
1 teaspoon canola oil

1. Mix the cold water and vinegar into the dry mustard to make a thick paste.

2. Mix in the roasted garlic and the oil until very smooth.

3. Allow the mustard to sit for thirty minutes before serving to meld the flavors.

Soups

Mustard adds a little something extra to any soup. There is even a recipe here for soup made with mustard greens.

Old-Style Mustard Soup

Mustard soup? It may sound a little strange, but wait until you taste it. You won't believe how good it is.

YIELD: 6 SERVINGS
¼ cup cornstarch
1 tablespoon dry mustard powder
5 cups strong beef bouillon
1 cup beer (optional) (if not using beer, use a total of 6 cups bouillon)
Salt and pepper to taste
4 green onions, tops included, finely chopped
¼ cup cooked ham, finely chopped

1. In a large soup pot, combine cornstarch and mustard. Add a little cold water, and stir to make a smooth paste.

2. Gradually stir in the bouillon, stirring constantly to make sure the mixture stays smooth. Stir in the beer and salt and pepper.

3. Cook over medium heat, stirring constantly, until the mixture boils and thickens. Reduce the heat and simmer for a few minutes, stirring often.

4. Ladle the soup into bowls, and scatter bits of green onion and ham on top. Serve immediately.

Hearty Mustard Soup

Try this soup as the centerpiece of a quick Sunday night supper.
Put a sandwich on the side, or serve with Quick
Fiesta Cornbread (see page 196).

YIELD: 6 SERVINGS

2 large potatoes, peeled and diced

3 medium onions, peeled and diced

4 cups beef bouillon

1 tablespoon dry mustard powder

2 tablespoons cold water

Salt and pepper to taste

1. In a soup pot, cook the potatoes and onion in the beef bouillon until the vegetables are very tender. Drain, reserving liquid.

2. Mash the potatoes and onions together by hand. Aim for a smooth texture, but not a purée.

3. Pour the reserved liquid over the vegetables and continue cooking. Stirring constantly, bring the soup back to a simmer.

4. Add the cold water to the mustard, and stir to form a paste.

5. Add the mustard paste to the soup, stirring well to combine.

6. Taste. Add salt and pepper as needed.

Artichoke Soup With Rock Shrimp and Mustard Cream

Chef Bob Hurley of the Napa Valley Grille prepared this soup
at the Napa Valley Mustard Festival in 1998. It was served to great
applause. This is definitely not the soup for a soup-and-sandwich
supper. Serve this intensely flavorful soup as an elegant
appetizer for your next dinner party. Enjoy.

YIELD: 10 SERVINGS

10 cups chicken stock
6 medium artichokes
1 bunch fresh sage
2 large onions, peeled and chopped
4 large leeks, split, washed, and trimmed of green
3 ounces smoked turkey bacon, diced
8 cloves garlic, peeled
8 ounces whole butter
3 medium potatoes, peeled and diced
2 cups rock shrimp
Salt and pepper to taste
MUSTARD CREAM
$\frac{1}{2}$ pint fresh heavy cream
1 tablespoon whole-grain mustard

1. In a large pot, bring the chicken stock and artichokes to a boil. Cook for thirty minutes.

2. Remove the artichokes, and separate the bottoms from the leaves. Return the leaves to the stock, and continue cooking for another 20 minutes.

3. While the stock cooks, cook sage, onions, leeks, bacon, garlic, and butter in another large pot over low heat until the onions are translucent and the bacon is limp and partially rendered.

4. Strain stock and add to the vegetable mixture.

5. Add the potatoes, and cook for approximately twenty minutes, or until the potatoes are very soft.

6. Put the soup into a blender or food processor, and purée.

7. Put the puréed soup back into the pot and bring to a boil. When the soup is boiling, add the rock shrimp. Season with salt and pepper to taste.

8. Prepare the mustard cream by whisking the heavy cream until thick, but not whipped. Whisk in the whole-grain mustard.

9. Ladle the soup into bowls, and top with a generous dollop of mustard cream. Serve immediately.

Creamy Mustard Green Soup

A bowlful of this creamy soup complemented with a sandwich makes a perfect family lunch or easy Sunday supper. It can also serve as the first course at a formal dinner party. It's a sure-fire conversation starter, too.

YIELD: 6 SERVINGS

3 cups (packed) mustard greens, washed and torn into small pieces

6 cups nonfat milk

I cup mashed potatoes

5 tablespoons butter (no substitutions)

I cup Monterey jack cheese, grated

Salt and pepper to taste

I cup nonfat sour cream

1. In a blender, purée the torn greens with about one cup of the milk.

2. Pour the purée into a large saucepan, and add the rest of the milk and all ingredients except the sour cream.

3. Simmer over very low heat until the cheese is melted.

4. Remove from heat, and stir in the sour cream. If necessary, reheat gently. Serve immediately.

Hearty Salads

A hearty salad can be the foundation of an informal buffet or the making of a summer picnic. Be warned that some of these recipes call for mayonnaise, which contains eggs. If you use regular mayonnaise, remember that egg-based foods have the potential to build harmful bacteria when they are out of the refrigerator for too long. Just be sure you have a cooler that will keep mayonnaise-based salads very cold if you're carrying a basket to the park.

Basic Potato Salad

This potato salad would add the perfect touch
to any barbecue or picnic.

YIELD: 6–8 SERVINGS

$\frac{1}{4}$ cup olive oil or nonfat mayonnaise
1 tablespoon of your favorite prepared mustard
1 tablespoon lemon juice
$\frac{1}{2}$ teaspoon Tabasco sauce
2 tablespoons fresh dill, minced; or 2 teaspoons dried dill
1 clove garlic, crushed (optional)
$\frac{1}{4}$ teaspoon salt
Cracked black pepper to taste
1 pound red skin potatoes (with skins)

1. Combine all dressing ingredients, and whisk to blend. Set aside.

2. Cook the potatoes until tender, and dice them while hot.

3. Drizzle the potatoes with the dressing, and toss to combine. Refrigerate.

4. Add other ingredients to the potato salad, such as onion, hard-boiled egg, radish, green pepper, jalapeño pepper, pickle, and olives, if you desire.

No-Mayo Cole Slaw

Tote this full-flavored slaw to your next picnic. Expect applause.
Like all salads, it's best chilled, but you won't have to worry
if it has to sit on the table for a while because it
contains no mayonnaise.

YIELD: 6 SERVINGS

DRESSING

1 ½ teaspoons mustard
1 ½ teaspoons orange zest (when grating, avoid the bitter white membrane)
2 tablespoons orange juice
1 tablespoon apple cider vinegar
1 teaspoon caraway seeds
1 teaspoon celery seeds
½ teaspoon sugar
Salt and cracked pepper to taste
½ cup olive oil

VEGETABLES

8 cups shredded cabbage, red and white mixed
2 carrots, coarsely grated
2 peppers (green, red, or yellow), slivered

1. In a large bowl, whisk together the first 8 ingredients for the dressing.

2. Add the olive oil very slowly, whisking until the ingredients are well combined and the dressing is slightly thickened.

3. Add the vegetables, tossing to coat with dressing.

4. Refrigerate for at least 3 hours to allow the flavor to permeate the vegetables.

Cantonese Chicken Salad

Here's another version of a Chinese chicken salad.
This recipe makes a delicious one-dish meal.

YIELD: 4 SERVINGS
I chicken breast, slivered
2 julienne carrots
I small onion, thinly sliced and separated into circles
I 9-ounce package frozen French green beans, thawed and drained
I 8-ounce can sliced water chestnuts, drained
DRESSING
⅓ cup oyster sauce
I tablespoon sesame oil
I tablespoon hot Chinese mustard (see page 114 for a recipe)
I tablespoon rice vinegar

1. Arrange chicken slivers and carrot sticks in steamer and cover. If you do not have a steamer, put the items in a colander or strainer. Place the colander or strainer over a pan with several inches of boiling water in it, and cover. Steam the chicken and carrot sticks over (not in) boiling water for 2 minutes.

2. Add the onion, green beans, and water chestnuts. Steam for another 2 minutes, or until the chicken is no longer pink and is fork-tender.

3. Put the cooked chicken and vegetables in a large bowl and set aside.

4. Put the dressing ingredients in a lidded jar. Shake well to combine.

5. Drizzle the dressing over the chicken and vegetables and toss, making sure all ingredients are coated with dressing.

6. Refrigerate for at least 2 hours before serving.

Warm Whole-Grain Mustard Potato Salad

This hearty salad is one of the original mustard recipes introduced at the Napa Valley Mustard Festival in 1998. Credit goes to Andrew Sutton, Executive Chef of Auberge du Soleil. Chef Sutton serves this salad with grilled smoked duck sausage.

YIELD: 4 SERVINGS
2 pounds Red Bliss potatoes (with skins)
2 ounces olive oil
I large julienne red onion
I ounce whole-grain mustard
2 ounces sherry vinegar
2 tablespoons chopped parsley
Salt and pepper to taste

1. Steam potatoes until tender. Chill immediately with ice.

2. When the potatoes are cool, carefully quarter them, leaving the skin intact.

3. Heat the olive oil in a large sauté pan over low heat. Sauté the onion until tender and translucent. Do not let it brown.

4. Add the potatoes and salt and pepper, and toss gently.

5. Add mustard, sherry vinegar, and parsley. Toss gently.

6. Serve while still warm.

White Bean Salad

This lightly dressed but zesty bean salad and the Black Bean Salad on page 125 are welcome additions to a buffet or a light family meal.

YIELD: 6–8 SERVINGS

1 19-ounce can of white beans, drained and rinsed
$\frac{1}{2}$ cup flat-leaf parsley, coarsely chopped
$\frac{1}{4}$ cup mint, finely chopped (optional)
2 cloves garlic, finely chopped
$\frac{1}{8}$ cup onion, finely chopped
2 tablespoons lemon juice
2 tablespoons water
1 tablespoon honey
$\frac{1}{2}$ tablespoon of your favorite prepared mustard
$\frac{1}{4}$ teaspoon salt
Cracked pepper to taste

1. Toss the beans with the chopped ingredients in a large bowl until well combined.

2. In a small bowl, mix the remaining ingredients together.

3. Drizzle the dressing over the bean mixture, and toss gently to coat.

4. Serve immediately.

Black Bean Salad

*Try this salad as an alternative to the White Bean Salad
on page 124.*

YIELD: 6–8 SERVINGS
1 19-ounce can black beans, drained and rinsed
2 cloves garlic, finely chopped
$\frac{1}{8}$ cup onion, finely chopped
2 tablespoons fresh cilantro, coarsely chopped
1 jalapeño pepper, finely chopped (optional)
2 tablespoons lime juice
2 tablespoons water
1 tablespoon honey
$\frac{1}{2}$ tablespoon of your favorite prepared mustard
$\frac{1}{4}$ teaspoon salt
Cracked pepper to taste

1. Toss the beans with the chopped ingredients in a large bowl until well combined.

2. In a small bowl, mix the remaining ingredients together to make a dressing.

3. Drizzle the dressing over the bean mixture, and toss gently to coat.

4. Serve immediately.

Variation: If you're looking for a zippy dip for a party, just blend the ingredients for this salad or the White Bean Salad on page 124 in a food processor. Voila! White Bean Dip or Black Bean Dip. Serve with crunchy tortilla chips.

Salad-in-a-Sandwich

This sandwich is a good start for a pool party or poker party,
or for watching the big game. Add some crunchy
tortilla chips, put out a bowl of salsa, and relax.

YIELD: 4 SERVINGS

I 12–14-inch round loaf of hearty bread
SPREAD
½ cup pitted black olives
I small clove roasted garlic, crushed
I tablespoon olive oil
I tablespoon lemon juice
I tablespoon basil leaves, finely chopped
SAUCE
2 tablespoons olive oil
I teaspoon apple cider vinegar
½ teaspoon of your favorite prepared mustard
Salt and cracked pepper to taste
4 ripe Roma tomatoes, diced
2 green onions, minced
FILLING
6 thin slices smoked ham
6 thin slices of dry salami (optional)
6 thin slices provolone cheese
2 cups salad greens, coarsely slivered

1. Prepare the loaf by cutting it in half horizontally. Remove the center of the bread from both halves, leaving about 2 inches of bread all around.

2. Prepare the spread by combining all of the ingredients in a food processor and pulsing until smooth. Set aside.

3. Prepare the sauce by whisking the oil, vinegar, mustard, and salt and pepper together in a large bowl. When well combined, stir in the tomatoes and green onions. Set aside.

4. Cover the inside of each half of the bread with the spread.

5. Line the dressed bottom half of the bread with half the slivered greens.

6. Put half the sauce on top of the greens.

7. Layer the meat and cheese over the dressed greens, arranging the slices to fit.

8. Dress with the remaining sauce, then top with the remaining greens.

9. Fit the top half of the bread over the filled bottom half.

10. Wrap with foil. Top this creation with a plate and weight it down with something heavy to press the ingredients together. Refrigerate. This salad-sandwich will hold nicely as long as overnight, but it needs at least an hour in the refrigerator to meld the flavors of all of the ingredients.

11. To serve, cut into fourths.

Basic Egg Salad

For a fine family lunch or quick supper, have this egg salad
on a sandwich with a steaming bowl of soup.
Also, try it as a stuffing for tomatoes.

YIELD: 4 SERVINGS
1/4 cup nonfat mayonnaise
I green onion minced, top included
1/2 teaspoon of your favorite prepared mustard
1/2 teaspoon celery salt
Cracked pepper to taste
4 hard-cooked eggs

1. Mix all ingredients but eggs together well to make a dressing.

2. Dice the eggs and add to the dressing. Mix well with a fork, mashing the eggs slightly.

Basic Cole Slaw

This quick and easy cole slaw is definitely a crowd-pleaser.

YIELD: 6–8 SERVINGS

1 tablespoon of your favorite prepared mustard
1 teaspoon sugar
$1/4$ cup apple cider vinegar
$1/2$ cup nonfat mayonnaise
3 cups shredded red and white cabbage

1. Combine mustard, sugar, vinegar, and mayonnaise. Whisk to blend.

2. Toss the cabbage with the dressing.

3. Refrigerate for at least one hour before serving to allow the flavors to blend.

4. Try adding $1/2$ cup shredded carrots and $1/4$ cup raisins to the salad before refrigerating.

Orange Cup

These colorful little fruit salad cups are excellent served alongside cold meats and are a tasty addition to a buffet table.

YIELD: 4 SERVINGS

2 oranges
1 apple
12 red seedless grapes
4 tablespoons Fruity Vinaigrette Dressing (see recipe on page 134)
Nonfat sour cream or nonfat vanilla yogurt

1. Cut the oranges in half. Each half will be used as a serving cup.

2. Scoop out the fruit as cleanly as possible. Remove the white membrane from the orange sections, and cut each section into pieces. Put the cut oranges in a medium-sized bowl.

3. Dice the apple, leaving the peel on, and toss with the orange pieces. Add the grapes.

4. Toss the fruit with the dressing.

5. Spoon equal amounts of the dressed fruit into each orange cup.

6. Top with a spoonful of nonfat sour cream or vanilla yogurt.

Chinese Chicken Salad

Many people use Chinese chicken salad as the centerpiece of the meal. That's the way we like it at my house. Fried won tons or steamed dim sum are perfect accompaniments.

YIELD: 4–6 SERVINGS

2 cooked skinless chicken breasts, cooled and shredded

5 cups (packed) shredded lettuce

3/4 cup green onions minced (tops included)

1/2 cup chopped cilantro (optional)

DRESSING

1/2 cup rice vinegar

3 tablespoons sugar

1/2 teaspoon dry mustard powder

2 tablespoons soy sauce

1 tablespoon sesame oil

1. Combine the shredded chicken, lettuce, onions, and cilantro in a large bowl.

2. Prepare the dressing by combining all ingredients in a lidded jar. Shake until the sugar and mustard dissolve.

3. Pour the dressing over fixings, and toss well. Serve immediately.

Celeriac-Mustard Salad

Celeriac, also known as celery root, is prized in Europe, where it is used in dishes we celebrate as "continental cuisine." Celeriac is a cousin of common celery, but it is cultivated for its bulbous root. The stalks are not used. With its yogurt base, this cool and refreshing salad has real continental flavor.

YIELD: 4 SERVINGS

1 tablespoon of your favorite prepared mustard
1 tablespoon lemon juice
$\frac{1}{4}$ cup plain yogurt
2 medium scrubbed, peeled, julienne celeriac roots
2 tablespoons green onions or chives, finely chopped
2 tablespoons flat-leaf parsley, finely chopped

1. Combine the mustard, lemon juice, and yogurt in a medium-sized bowl. Set aside.

2. Add the celeriac to the mustard mixture, stirring well to coat all the strips. Cover and marinate for at least 3 hours. Marinate it overnight in the refrigerator, if you wish.

3. When ready to serve, add the chopped greens, and toss to combine.

4. For a nice presentation, mound this salad on a plate lined with crunchy radicchio leaves.

Salad Dressings

No matter how fresh and crisp the greens, vegetables, and fruits may be, almost everyone will agree that a salad is improved with a flavorful dressing. This section provides a great selection. You may also use any of these dressings on a pasta salad or roasted vegetables.

Gourmet Mustard-Seed-Infused Olive Oil

This infused oil makes a dazzling hostess gift. Pour the oil into a decorative bottle, cap it, and tie several lengths of raffia around the top. Wrap the oil in a checked linen napkin, and nestle it in a basket. Add a loaf of crusty bread and a bottle of good wine, and off you go to a weekend house party. This gourmet oil can also be the basis for a delicious vinaigrette, but it's so good that you'll enjoy it simply drizzled on crusty bread. The next time you're serving an Italian feast, forget the garlic toast. Provide crusty bread and pass a cruet of infused olive oil for dipping and drizzling. You'll get raves.

YIELD: 17 OUNCES
1 17-ounce bottle of olive oil
1 tablespoon mustard seed
$\frac{1}{2}$ tablespoon peppercorns
A sprig of fresh rosemary
$\frac{1}{2}$ clove garlic

1. Pour 3 ounces of the olive oil into a separate container to prevent overflow when all ingredients are added. Set aside.
2. Crack the mustard seed and peppercorns and drop them and the garlic and rosemary into the bottle of oil.
3. Add enough reserved oil to top off the bottle.
4. Cap the bottle and let the oil rest in a dark place for 5 to 7 days. Remove the rosemary and garlic.
5. To serve, strain the oil into a cruet.

Basic Mustard Salad Dressing

This dressing is particularly good over spinach or mustard greens,
but it's equally tasty tossed with mixed greens. If you don't use
it all, refrigerate the remainder in a sealed container.

YIELD: 1 ½ CUPS
3 tablespoons white vinegar
2 tablespoons lemon juice
2 teaspoons mustard
1 teaspoon sugar
1 teaspoon salt
1 cup olive oil

1. Combine the first 5 ingredients in a small bowl, and whisk together.
2. Drizzle in the oil very slowly, whisking well until the dressing thickens. If you prefer, you may use a blender to insure that the dressing doesn't separate on standing.

Fast Mustard Vinaigrette

This vinaigrette is quick, easy, and oh-so good.

YIELD: ¾ CUP
½ cup olive oil
3 tablespoons vinegar
1 tablespoon of your favorite prepared mustard
½ teaspoon salt
⅛ teaspoon cayenne or Tabasco sauce (optional)

1. Combine all ingredients in a jar with a tight lid, and mix well. Refrigerate.
2. Shake well before serving.

Easy Honey-Mustard Vinaigrette

This dressing is as wonderful with fruit as it is with greens.

YIELD: ³/₄ CUP

½ cup olive oil

3 tablespoons apple cider vinegar

I tablespoon honey mustard

I teaspoon honey

½ teaspoon salt (optional)

1. Combine all ingredients in a jar with a tight lid, and mix well. Refrigerate.

2. Shake well before serving.

Hearty Mustard Vinaigrette

This dressing stands up well to any hearty salad, especially one that includes chicken or other meats.

YIELD: ¼ CUP

I teaspoon Dijon-style mustard

I tablespoon balsamic vinegar

½ teaspoon minced garlic, crushed

½ teaspoon dried basil, crushed

3 tablespoons olive oil

Salt and cracked pepper to taste

1. Combine mustard, vinegar, garlic, and basil in a small bowl.

2. Whisk in olive oil.

3. Season with salt and pepper to taste.

Fruity Vinaigrette

Enjoy this dressing over a few of your favorite fresh fruits cut into bite-sized pieces.

YIELD: ³/₄ CUP
¹/₄ cup olive oil
2 tablespoons raspberry or red wine vinegar
3 tablespoons orange juice
2 teaspoons lemon juice
¹/₂ tablespoon of your favorite prepared mustard
3 teaspoons honey
I teaspoon fresh ginger, grated (optional)
¹/₈ teaspoon salt
Cracked black pepper to taste

1. Combine all ingredients in a jar with a tight lid.

2. Shake well and refrigerate.

3. Shake well before serving.

Sassy Mustard Dressing

This well-flavored dressing is especially good with roasted vegetables.

YIELD: ¹/₄ CUP
¹/₄ cup olive oil
3 tablespoons white wine vinegar
I tablespoon lemon juice
I teaspoon prepared mustard
I clove garlic, crushed
¹/₄ teaspoon cayenne pepper or Tabasco sauce
¹/₄ teaspoon salt
Cracked black pepper to taste

I. Combine all ingredients in a jar with a tight lid and mix well. Refrigerate.

2. Shake well before serving.

3. For intense flavor, prepare this dressing 2 days before serving.

Tarragon Mustard Dressing

This hearty dressing is excellent with a chef's salad. Prepare a salad of strong mixed greens that includes romaine and endive. Add alfalfa sprouts, slivers of red onion, ripe cherry tomatoes (halved), hard-cooked egg, and strips of cooked white-meat chicken or turkey. Drizzle on the dressing, and toss gently.

YIELD: $1/4$ CUP
$1/4$ cup olive oil
3 tablespoons tarragon vinegar
2 teaspoons tarragon mustard
I tablespoon finely chopped fresh tarragon (or I teaspoon dried)
$1/4$ teaspoon salt
Cracked black pepper to taste

Combine all ingredients in a jar with a tight lid. Shake well and refrigerate.

Sauces

These sauces can dress up many dishes, including meat, fish, and steamed or roasted vegetables, and many are essential on sandwiches. They can be served hot or cold. Some sauces have a strong mustard flavor, while others bring barely a hint of mustard's pungency to the dish.

Hurry-up Barbecue Sauce

There are so many varieties of barbecue sauce on the market nowadays that everyone buys it instead of making it. However, the time may come when you want to barbecue, but you're out of prepared barbecue sauce, and it's too much trouble to go to the store. Here's the quick-fix solution for barbecued chicken or pork, made with ingredients you have on hand. This sauce is especially good if you're cooking on the outdoor grill, but it is also excellent for oven-barbecued meats.

YIELD: ABOUT 1 ½ CUPS

I tablespoon canola oil
¼ cup chopped onions
½ cup water
2 tablespoons vinegar
2 tablespoons brown sugar
I cup ketchup or chili sauce
I tablespoon Worcestershire sauce
I tablespoon of your favorite prepared mustard
¼ cup lemon juice

1. Sauté the onions in the oil in a saucepan until nicely browned.

2. Add the other ingredients. Mix well to combine.

3. Simmer the sauce for about 20 minutes.

4. Baste meat several times during cooking with this sweet and tangy sauce.

Grandma's Rich Cheese Sauce

*This is the mouth-watering, luscious old-fashioned cheese sauce
we all remember with such pleasure.*

YIELD: 1 ½ CUPS

I cup evaporated milk

8 ounces grated cheddar cheese

½ teaspoon of your favorite prepared mustard

I teaspoon salt

¼ teaspoon paprika

¼ teaspoon cayenne pepper (optional)

1. Heat the milk in a medium-sized heavy saucepan over very low heat until it begins to simmer.

2. Add the grated cheese and cook, stirring constantly, until the cheese melts and the sauce is smooth.

3. Stir in the mustard and seasonings.

4. Serve hot over vegetables, including potatoes, or make a quick macaroni-and-cheese dinner by stirring the sauce into 4 cups of cooked elbow macaroni.

Easy Fat-Free Mustard Sauce

*This fast and easy mustard sauce is good for dipping vegetables
and makes a tasty sandwich spread as well.*

YIELD: 6 TABLESPOONS

4 tablespoons fat-free mayonnaise

2 tablespoons of your favorite prepared mustard

Mix the mayonnaise and mustard together in a small bowl ten minutes before serving. The delay allows the full flavor of the mustard to permeate the mayonnaise.

Sweet and Sour Mustard Sauce

*This sauce tastes good with all meats, especially chicken and turkey.
It's great for dressing up leftovers, too. For a surprise treat, try
serving this sauce over plain rice.*

YIELD: 1 1/2 CUPS

1 tablespoon cornstarch
1 cup chicken or vegetable broth
1 teaspoon apple cider vinegar
3 tablespoons of the prepared mustard of your choice
2 tablespoons honey

1. Gradually add the broth to the cornstarch, stirring until smooth.

2. Add the rest of the ingredients and combine well.

3. Simmer over low heat, stirring constantly, until thickened—
about 5 minutes.

Easy Fat-Free Tartar Sauce

*This tartar sauce is just as tasty as regular tartar sauce—
but it's fat-free! You'll never know the difference.*

YIELD: 1 CUP

3/4 cup fat-free sour cream or fat-free mayonnaise
2 tablespoons chopped pickle of your choice
1 tablespoon grated onion or finely chopped chives
1/4 cup chopped olives
1/2 tablespoon of your favorite prepared mustard
1 tablespoon fresh tarragon or 1 teaspoon dried tarragon

Combine all ingredients well. Serve chilled.

Old-Style Cooked Tartar Sauce

*If British pub-food is your idea of heaven, you may fancy
an occasional feast of calorie-laden, fat-saturated, English-style
deep-fried fish and chips, with a sprinkle of malt vinegar on your
chips. The traditional accompaniment is a heaping helping of tartar
sauce. Of course, we all know that steamed or poached fish is a much
healthier choice, but there's no reason to forego the tartar sauce if
you're counting calories and fat grams. Try this traditional
tartar sauce just like grandmother used to make.*

YIELD: 2 CUPS
$\frac{1}{3}$ cup flour
I cup stock or bouillon
2 egg yolks or $\frac{1}{2}$ cup egg substitute
I cup olive oil
I tablespoon vinegar
I teaspoon of your favorite prepared mustard
I cup pickle relish of your choice
$\frac{1}{4}$ teaspoon salt (optional)

1. In a medium saucepan, add the stock very slowly to the flour, mixing until smooth. Stirring constantly, cook these ingredients over low heat until they thicken. Remove from heat.

2. Very slowly beat in the egg yolks or substitute and oil.

3. Continue beating while adding the remaining ingredients.

4. Chill and serve cold.

Spicy Low-Cal Cheese Sauce

This sauce is wonderful over steamed cauliflower or broccoli.

YIELD: 1 $\frac{1}{2}$ CUPS
2 tablespoons butter (do not use substitutes)
2 tablespoons flour
1 $\frac{1}{2}$ cups nonfat milk
1 cup nonfat or low-fat grated cheddar cheese
$\frac{1}{2}$ teaspoon prepared mustard
$\frac{1}{4}$ teaspoon Tabasco sauce
$\frac{1}{2}$ teaspoon salt
$\frac{1}{8}$ teaspoon paprika

1. Melt the butter in a medium saucepan, and stir in the flour.

2. When mixed well, slowly add the milk.

3. When the sauce is smooth and simmering, add the grated cheese.

4. When the cheese is melted, add the mustard and seasonings.

5. Serve hot.

Hot Honey Mustard Sauce

*Try this cheese-free sauce over steamed vegetables,
such as broccoli, cauliflower, or asparagus.*

YIELD: ABOUT 1 CUP
$\frac{1}{2}$ cup nonfat mayonnaise
$\frac{1}{4}$ cup honey
$\frac{1}{4}$ cup prepared mustard
$\frac{1}{4}$ cup lemon juice

In a medium-sized saucepan, combine all ingredients and mix well.
Place over low heat. Cook until the sauce is hot, stirring constantly.

Asian Mayonnaise

*This healthy mayonnaise works equally well as a sauce or
sandwich spread, and it's especially good with fish.*

YIELD: I CUP
I cup crumbled tofu
2 tablespoons vinegar
I tablespoon olive oil
I teaspoon mustard
I teaspoon lemon juice
$\frac{1}{2}$ teaspoon tamari

Put all ingredients in a blender. Process on low speed until smooth
and creamy.

Old-Style Mustard Cream Sauce

*Try this mustard sauce over plants from the "Brassica" family,
such as cauliflower and broccoli.*

YIELD: $\frac{1}{2}$ CUP
$\frac{1}{2}$ cup thick cream
2 teaspoons of your favorite prepared mustard
$\frac{1}{4}$ teaspoon salt
$\frac{1}{8}$ teaspoon paprika

1. Combine all of the ingredients in a small heavy saucepan.

2. Stirring constantly, cook the sauce over very low heat until it
thickens. Do not allow it to boil.

3. Serve hot over vegetables.

Easy No-Cook Old-Style Tartar Sauce

For a quick, easy tartar sauce, try this one.

YIELD: 1 CUP
1 teaspoon Dijon-style mustard
1 teaspoon confectioners' sugar
$\frac{1}{4}$ teaspoon salt
$\frac{1}{8}$ teaspoon pepper
$\frac{1}{2}$ cup egg substitute
$\frac{1}{2}$ cup olive oil
3 tablespoons vinegar
2 tablespoons finely chopped sweet, dill, or bread-and-butter pickles
1 tablespoon capers (optional)
1 tablespoon finely chopped olives of your choice (optional)

1. Combine the first 5 ingredients in a small bowl and beat well. Set aside.

2. Mix the olive oil and vinegar together. Add the mustard mixture very slowly to the oil and vinegar, beating until thick.

3. When the sauce is thickened, add the pickles, capers, and olives.

4. Chill, and serve cold.

Rémoulade Sauce

Try serving a spoonful of this classic New Orleans favorite drizzled on cold sliced turkey or chicken. It's also excellent with fish or shellfish.

YIELD: I CUP

I cup fat-free mayonnaise
2 tablespoons fresh parsley, finely chopped
I tablespoon dill pickle, finely chopped
2 teaspoons Dijon-style mustard
$\frac{1}{2}$ teaspoon apple cider vinegar
$\frac{1}{2}$ teaspoon Worcestershire sauce
$\frac{1}{2}$ teaspoon dried tarragon, crumbled
I teaspoon capers, rinsed and finely chopped (optional)

1. In a medium-sized bowl, combine all ingredients. Mix well.

2. Allow the sauce to stand refrigerated for 30 minutes to meld flavors.

Marinades

A marinade is a combination of oil and an acidic liquid, such as vinegar or wine, well-seasoned with herbs and spices. Marinades are used as steeping liquid to tenderize a tough cut of meat or to add flavor to meats, fish, and vegetables prior to cooking. If you choose to use wine in place of vinegar, be sure to use a wine that's acceptable for drinking. It doesn't have to be an expensive vintage, and either red or white is fine, but it must be palatable. Don't use cooking wine, which contains sodium. Apple cider and plain white vinegar are both acceptable, but you can use a gourmet vinegar, if you prefer. Because of the acid content of marinades, it's necessary to keep them in a non-reactive container, such as glass or plastic. Plastic bags work well.

Full-Flavored Marinade

This delicious marinade will add flavor to any meats or vegetables. Try it as an alternative to the Basic Marinade.

YIELD: 2 1/2 CUPS

2 cups vinegar or wine
1/2 cup olive oil
1 small onion, grated
2 garlic cloves, minced or crushed
1 teaspoon of your favorite prepared mustard
2 teaspoons Worcestershire sauce
1 teaspoon Tabasco sauce
1 teaspoon cracked pepper

1. Combine all ingredients in a large bowl.

2. Use to marinate meat or vegetables (follow the directions on page 145).

Basic Meat Marinade

This basic marinade will make your meats tender and delicious. Try it the next time you make a rump roast or almost any meat.

Yield: 2 ½ cups

2 cups vinegar or wine
½ cup olive oil
1 small onion, grated
1 teaspoon of your favorite prepared mustard
1 teaspoon cracked pepper

1. Combine all ingredients.

2. Follow the directions below for marinating meat.

Marinating Meat and Vegetables

Using marinades is easy. To tenderize a tough cut of meat, such as a rump roast or stewing meat, pour the marinade over the meat in a plastic bag. Seal and refrigerate. Allow the meat to steep for four hours, or even overnight. Turn the meat several times to insure that all surfaces come in contact with the marinade. Remove the meat from the marinade and cook as desired. After marinating meat, discard the marinade. A marinade that has been in contact with raw meat contains blood and bacteria. It should not be used as a base for gravy or sauce.

If making vegetables, marinate them for one hour. Roast marinated vegetables, such as peppers (all kinds), portabella or shiitake mushrooms, whole Italian tomatoes, and small redskin potatoes (with skins), in an oven preheated to 350°F for 30 to 40 minutes, or until tender.

Honey-Mustard Marinade

*This light marinade is excellent for chicken or pork,
especially if you're planning on grilling.*

YIELD: I CUP
$\frac{1}{3}$ cup olive oil
$\frac{1}{3}$ cup orange juice
$\frac{1}{4}$ cup honey mustard
3 tablespoons honey
$\frac{3}{4}$ teaspoon dried thyme, crumbled
2 cloves garlic, minced (optional)

1. Combine all ingredients in a large bowl.

2. Follow the marinating directions on page 145.

Pickles and Relishes

Pickles are foods that have been salted or steeped in brine, which is a mixture of salt and water, before being preserved in a highly flavored vinegar and sugar-based liquid. Pickling spice, available at any supermarket, is a spicy and delicious combination of dill, fenugreek, mustard seeds, celery seeds, black pepper, red pepper, cloves, allspice, ginger, bay leaves, and cumin. Yes, I know. It's much easier to buy prepared pickles and relishes at the grocery store. But they're not as much trouble to prepare as you might think, and they are fun to make. This chapter gives you several pickle and relish recipes "like grandma used to make," including pickles made with olive oil. All are delicious.

Mustard Refrigerator Pickles

These pickles are both easy to make and good to eat.

YIELD: 50 PICKLES
50 small (4-inch) washed cucumbers
I gallon apple cider vinegar
3 cups sugar
I tablespoon mustard seed (any type)
$\frac{1}{2}$ cup coarse salt (not iodized)

1. Cut off the stems of the cucumbers, and quarter them lengthwise. Place them in a 3-gallon crock.

2. Combine the remaining ingredients. Stir the mixture until the sugar and salt are well dissolved.

3. Pour the vinegar mixture over the cucumbers. Cover with a plate. To keep the cucumbers immersed in the liquid, place a plate on top and put a weight on the plate. Refrigerate.

4. Permit the pickles to ripen for 4 to 7 days before serving.

Mixed Mustard Pickles

My grandmother's mustard pickles were always the hit of the picnic.

YIELD: 4–6 QUARTS
I cup coarse salt (not iodized)
2 quarts water
I pound small green washed cucumbers
I pound green beans cut into bite-sized pieces
6–8 green tomatoes
I head of cauliflower broken into florets
12 small pearl onions
I $\frac{1}{2}$ cups flour
6 tablespoons dry mustard powder
I $\frac{1}{2}$ tablespoons turmeric
10 cups apple cider vinegar
2 $\frac{1}{2}$ cups sugar
3 tablespoons celery seed

1. Prepare a brine by dissolving the salt in the water in a large saucepan. Heat to boiling.

2. In a large bowl, cover the cucumber slices with the hot brine, and let them marinate for twelve hours.

3. Drain and rinse the cucumber slices. Set aside.

4. Blanch the vegetables by plunging them into enough boiling lightly salted water to cover them. When the water begins to boil, permit the vegetables to cook for 2 minutes. Drain well.

5. In a large bowl combine the vegetables with the cucumber slices and add onions. Set aside.

6. Combine the flour, dry mustard, and turmeric. Slowly add 2 cups of the vinegar and stir until smooth.

7. Combine the sugar with the remaining 8 cups of vinegar in a large saucepan and bring to a boil.

8. Stirring constantly, add the flour mixture to the sauce, and return to boiling point.

9. When the sauce is smooth and boiling, pour it over the drained vegetables.

10. Place the pickles and their liquid in hot sterilized jars. Seal according to the manufacturer's instructions.

11. Allow the pickles to ripen for 3 weeks before serving.

Mustard Pickles With Olive Oil

This is an interesting and delicious variation on the traditional pickles.

YIELD: 24 PICKLES
24 small washed cucumbers, 3 to 4 inches long
½ cup coarse salt (not iodized)
2 small onions
4 cups cider vinegar
½ cup olive oil
I cup mustard seed (preferably white)
I tablespoon celery seed

1. Cut the cucumbers into thin $1/_8$-inch-thick circles.

2. Sprinkle the cucumbers with salt, and let them sit for three hours. Drain off any accumulated juices, and pat the cucumbers dry with a paper towel.

3. Peel the onions, and slice them very thinly. Add the onions to the drained cucumber slices.

4. Combine the remaining ingredients, and mix thoroughly.

5. Place the cucumbers and onions in sterilized jars, and fill with the liquid. Refrigerate.

6. Permit the pickles to ripen for 3 weeks before serving.

Cranberry-Raisin Pickle

*Pickles such as these are an important part of the meal in India.
Dress up steamed rice, rice pilaf, and a traditional Indian curry
by serving a spoonful of pickle on the side of the plate. If you decide
to depart from the traditional cranberry sauce and surprise your
Thanksgiving guests with this sweet and spicy pickled cranberry
relish, they should be warned that it's not for the timid.*

YIELD: 2 QUARTS
3 tablespoons pickle masala (see page 153)
4 tablespoons red wine vinegar
1 tablespoon salt
3 tablespoons mustard oil (see page 152)
1 teaspoon mustard seed
1 pound fresh cranberries, washed and dried
3 tablespoons julienne garlic
2 tablespoons julienne ginger root
2 chopped green chilies (optional)
$\frac{1}{4}$ cup raisins
2 tablespoons molasses

1. In a small bowl, make a paste of the masala, vinegar, and salt. Set aside.

2. Heat the mustard oil in a wok or skillet (not aluminum). When the oil is hot, sprinkle in the seeds and cover until the seeds pop. Add the garlic, ginger, and chilies, and stir until the garlic is lightly browned—about two or three minutes.

3. Add the cranberries and stir-fry until the berries start to crack open—about 5 minutes. Add the masala paste, and stir for one minute.

4. Remove from heat. Add the raisins and molasses and stir well. Let the pickle cool uncovered for 4 hours at room temperature.

5. Put the pickles into sterilized dry jars. Any excess moisture will spoil the pickles, so make sure the jars are dry. Seal the jars and let the pickles stand for at least one week before serving. Refrigerate after opening.

Green Mango Pickle

*I'm told that Green Mango Pickles are the most
popular pickles in India.*

YIELD: 10–12 SERVINGS

2 pounds firm green mangoes, washed, peeled, and cut into small cubes
1 tablespoon salt
3 tablespoons mustard oil (see page 152)
1 teaspoon mustard seed
3 tablespoons julienne garlic
2 tablespoons fresh julienne ginger root
3 chopped green chilies (optional)
3 tablespoons pickle masala
4 tablespoons white vinegar

1. In a medium-sized bowl, mix the mangoes with salt and cover. Set aside for at least 2 hours, but preferably overnight.

2. Heat the mustard oil in a wok or skillet (not aluminum) over medium heat. When the oil is hot, sprinkle in the mustard seeds, and cover until the seeds pop. Add the garlic, ginger, and chilies and stir until the garlic is lightly browned—about 2 or 3 minutes.

3. Mix the masala with the vinegar, making a paste, and add it to the skillet, stirring for one minute.

4. Stir the cubed mangoes into the other ingredients, and stir-fry for 2 minutes. Remove from the heat, and let the pickle cool uncovered for 4 hours at room temperature.

5. Put the pickles into sterilized dry jars. Any excess moisture will spoil the pickles, so make sure the jars are dry. Seal the jars, and let the pickles stand for at least one week before serving. Refrigerate after opening.

Egg Pickle of India

Pickled eggs are familiar to most of us, but I bet you've never had them this way. In India, this spicy egg pickle is used in salads or sandwiches.

YIELD: 6 EGGS
2 garlic cloves, slivered
$\frac{1}{2}$-inch piece ginger root, slivered
1 $\frac{1}{2}$ cups vinegar
$\frac{1}{2}$-inch piece of cinnamon stick
6 whole cloves
1 tablespoon cracked mustard seeds
6 peppercorns
3 mild red chilies
$\frac{1}{4}$ teaspoon sugar
Salt to taste
6 hard boiled eggs, shelled

1. Mash the garlic and ginger together.

2. Put all of the ingredients except the eggs in a saucepan, and bring to a fast simmer. Simmer for 15 minutes. Strain and cool the pickling liquid.

3. Put the shelled hardboiled eggs in a jar and pour the pickling liquid on top. Cover and refrigerate. Allow the eggs to remain in the liquid for 7 days.

Mustard Oil

When shopping for mustard oil, be sure to select a food-grade product. Some mustard oils are clearly marked "for massage use only." Look for a double-filtered mustard oil imported from India, where they cook with mustard oil regularly. Mustard oil seems mild at first acquaintance, but finishes with a fiery afterglow. Mustard oil can be found in stores that sell Indian foods. It's worth the trip.

Sweet Tomato Relish

This relish (or chutney, if you prefer) calls for panch phoron, a spicy blend of the spices of India that includes mustard seed, kalonji, fennel, fenugreek, and cumin. It is intensely flavorful but mild. This dish is wonderful with any meal, Indian or otherwise. Serve with steamed rice, rice pilaf, or curry. For a beautiful presentation, add the Indian Eggplant (see page 189) to the plate.

YIELD: 4–6 SERVINGS

2 tablespoons mustard oil (see page 152)
1 teaspoon panch phoron
1 tablespoon fresh ginger root, diced
1 pound firm tomatoes cut into wedges
1/4 cup sugar
1/2 teaspoon turmeric
1/2 teaspoon salt

1. In a wok or skillet, heat the mustard oil. Add the panch phoron and ginger. Stir to coat.

2. Add the tomatoes, sugar, turmeric, and salt and bring to a boil. Cook, stirring frequently until nicely thickened. This step will take about 10 minutes.

Pickle Masala

"Masala" simply means "mixture." The pickle masala of India is a fiery blend of powdered red chilies, turmeric, ginger, asafoetida (a resin obtained from the root of plants in the parsley family), mustard seeds, fenugreek, and dried green mangoes. The one I like best is from India's Spice 'n Flavor line. It's free of MSG, preservatives, and salt. It's a beautiful deep orange color, and it's very hot and spicy. Don't try smelling it. The masala is so fine that it will make you sneeze repeatedly. Pickle masala can be found at Indian groceries and other stores that sell Indian food.

Easy Mustard Relish

A spoonful of this relish will wake up any sandwich. Be sure to put out a bowlful when you're serving buffet-style, especially if the buffet includes an antipasto platter.

YIELD: ⅓ CUP
4 teaspoons coarsely grated (or finely chopped) onion
4 teaspoons coarsely grated (or finely chopped) green pepper
3 tablespoons mustard
3 teaspoons sugar
3 teaspoons olive oil
½ teaspoon cracked black pepper
3 teaspoons malt vinegar (optional)
I teaspoon horseradish (optional)

1. Combine all ingredients.

2. To permit the flavors to blend, allow the relish to "rest" for at least 30 minutes before serving.

Traditional Cucumber Pickles

These crunchy pickles are just like the ones Grandma always had on hand.

YIELD: 50 PICKLES
I cup coarse salt
3 quarts water
50 small washed cucumbers, about 2½ inches long
3 quarts apple cider vinegar
3 cups sugar
3 tablespoons pickling spice

1. Prepare a brine by dissolving the salt in 2 quarts of water in a large pot. Heat to boiling.

2. Cover the cucumbers with the hot brine in a large bowl. Let them marinate for 12 hours. Drain and rinse.

3. Combine vinegar, sugar, and pickling spice with 1 quart of water in a large pot to make a pickling syrup. Heat to boiling.

4. Place the cucumbers in hot sterilized jars. Fill with pickling syrup. Seal the jars according to the manufacturer's instructions.

5. Allow the pickles to ripen for three weeks before serving.

Easy Pickled Beets

*Pickled beets are always a treat. If you like pickled eggs, immerse
four shelled hard-boiled eggs in the liquid. These pretty pink
eggs can be quartered and served with the beets.
They're also nice sliced atop a salad.*

YIELD: 4–6 SERVINGS
1 can sliced beets
1 medium sweet red onion
2 tablespoons sugar
4 tablespoons olive oil
4 tablespoons vinegar
1 teaspoon mustard seeds

1. Drain the beets, and put them in a shallow bowl. Reserve the liquid.

2. Thinly slice the onion and toss the slices with the beets.

3. Mix the reserved liquid, sugar, oil, and vinegar together with a whisk. Add the mustard seeds.

4. Pour the liquid over the beets and onions. Toss to coat all surfaces with the spicy dressing. Cover and refrigerate overnight.

Meat and Poultry Entrées

When you're hungry, everything tastes good, but I think you'll agree that it tastes better when it's sauced with mustard. Nonetheless, mustard is much more than a sauce. This ancient herb is an essential ingredient in many dishes, as in Chicken Dijon, but why stop there? You'll find many other ways to use mustard with meat in this section. How about Bourbon Beef or Spicy Pork From India, and a few surprises, including Rabbit Saddle With Mustard Sauce?

Spicy Ham Spread

This recipe is a once- or twice-a-year favorite around our house. You can use your leftover Mustard-Glazed Baked Ham (see page 157) to make it. My family likes this sandwich spread on dark rye bread topped with crunchy butter lettuce. Extra mustard with the spread is a must at our house. Add a mixed-green or fruit salad, and you have a feast. It's also very good on crisp crackers.

YIELD 4 1/2 CUPS

2 cups cooked ham, very finely chopped
(If you have a meat grinder, grind the ham instead.)

4 tablespoons softened butter
(no substitutions)

4 teaspoons of your favorite prepared mustard

2 teaspoons honey

2 teaspoons brown sugar

1/4 teaspoon powdered cloves

Combine all ingredients in a food processor, and pulse until a smooth paste forms. A blender won't work. If you don't have a food processor, use a fork.

Mustard-Glazed Baked Ham

Because ham is so high in fat, I don't serve it more than once or twice a year. We reserve it for special occasions, and eat it sparingly. Some members of my family think this glaze is the best part. Scalloped potatoes just seem to go with ham. This makes a very rich dinner, so be sure to serve a salad of mixed greens lightly dressed with Fast Mustard Vinaigrette (see page 132). A thin, tart dressing will help cleanse and refresh the palate.

When you serve baked ham, you're bound to have leftovers. There's always sliced ham sandwiches, or macaroni and cheese with ham, or scalloped potatoes with ham, or ham salad.

YIELD: 10–12 SERVINGS
1 6–8-pound ham
Cloves
GLAZE
1 ½ cups dark brown sugar
⅓ cup finely crushed toasted bread crumbs
2 teaspoons dry mustard powder
4 tablespoons honey

1. Trim much of the fat from the ham, leaving just enough to score in the traditional diamond pattern.

2. Score the ham, stud it with whole cloves, and bake it until it's partially done—about 45 minutes—basting it several times with the pan juices.

3. Combine all of the ingredients for the glaze.

4. Bake the ham another 45 minutes. During this time, spread the glaze on the ham thickly. The glaze will be very thick. If it's too thick to spread, add a little more honey or very little water. The glaze will melt and crisp as the ham finishes cooking. Save enough to glaze the ham a second time.

Spicy Pork and Potatoes From India

*A lightly dressed green salad is the only accompaniment needed for
this dish. Fruit makes a perfect palate-cleansing finale.
Mango is a favorite fruit of India.*

YIELD: 4 SERVINGS
$\frac{1}{4}$ teaspoon turmeric
$\frac{1}{4}$ teaspoon cumin seeds
$\frac{1}{2}$-inch piece cinnamon stick
2 whole cloves
2 cardamom seeds
5 peppercorns
$\frac{1}{4}$ teaspoon mustard seeds
2 cloves of garlic, slivered
4 red chilies, slivered
2 green chilies, slivered
$\frac{1}{4}$ cup vinegar
1 tablespoon ginger root, grated
1 tablespoon clarified butter
3 medium onions, thinly sliced
1 pound pork steak, diced
Salt to taste
Water
2 pounds small potatoes, boiled, peeled, and diced

1. Toast the first 7 ingredients in a hot skillet over medium-high
heat until the spices are lightly browned.

2. Grind the toasted spices together with the garlic, chilies, vinegar,
and ginger. Set aside.

3. In a large skillet, melt the butter and sauté the onions until gold-
en. Add the diced pork steak, and stir in the spices.

4. Continue cooking the mixture until the pork is crisp and golden
in color.

5. Add enough water to cover, and simmer until the pork is tender and the gravy has thickened.

6. Add the diced potatoes, tossing to coat with the sauce. Continue cooking until the potatoes are heated through.

7. Serve in individual shallow bowls immediately.

Spicy Turkey Burgers

Just about everyone knows how to cook a hamburger, but many people don't want all that fat. You can still have burgers, if you're willing to make some sensible tradeoffs. In our household, we like quarter-pound turkey burgers. No, these burgers don't taste like hamburgers. They taste better. Try this on your family. Serve these burgers on toasted whole-wheat buns topped with shredded lettuce and thin-sliced rings of sweet red onion. We use a slathering of hot mustard in my house, but you can use nonfat mayonnaise and cheese, if you like.

YIELD: 4 SERVINGS
1 pound ground turkey
1/4 cup onion, finely minced
1/4 cup ketchup
1 tablespoon of your favorite prepared mustard
1/2 teaspoon salt
Cracked pepper to taste
Canola oil cooking spray

1. In a bowl, sprinkle the onion, ketchup, mustard, salt, and pepper over the ground turkey. Mix well, and form into four quarter-pound burgers.

2. Spray a frying pan with canola oil cooking spray, and preheat to medium heat. When the pan is hot, grill the burgers. Cook for about 5 to 7 minutes on each side, or until the meat is no longer pink.

Fricassee of Chicken
With Black-Eyed Peas

This low-calorie, fat-free stew combines white-meat chicken and hearty black-eyed peas with the sweet heat of mustard for an updated Southern-style favorite that the whole family will enjoy. Hot cornbread and a salad of mixed greens are the perfect accompaniments to this family dinner. Try the Quick Fiesta Cornbread (see page 196) with it. If black-eyed peas are not a usual dish in your household, please try this recipe. This hearty richly flavored fricassee will make you a convert.

YIELD: 8 SERVINGS

2 pounds of skinless chicken breasts,
rinsed and trimmed of visible fat

16-ounce can of black-eyed peas, rinsed and drained

2 cups water

2 tablespoons dry mustard powder

2 tablespoons brown sugar

1 large onion, coarsely chopped

1/4 cup fresh parsley

1. Coat a large frying pan with olive oil cooking spray. Place over medium-low heat. Pat the chicken dry with a paper towel and add to the heated pan. Brown lightly on all sides. Pour off and discard any fat that accumulates.

2. Add the remaining ingredients to the pan and mix well.

3. Cover and cook over medium heat for 45 minutes, or until the chicken is no longer pink on the inside.

Note: This dish cooks very nicely in a Crock-Pot, making it ideal for a busy-day meal. If using a Crock-Pot, put 1 cup dried black-eyed peas, rinsed and drained (do not use canned peas) in the pot. Sprinkle mustard powder, brown sugar, onion, and parsley over the peas. Place the lightly browned chicken pieces on top. Add just enough water to cover. Cook on low setting for 8 to 10 hours.

Creamy Coq au Vin
With Mustard and Mushrooms

*Here's another classic French dish, dressed up for a dinner party.
Indulge. This dish is so rich that I prefer to serve it with steamed
white rice and something green. Steamed broccoli and spinach
are both excellent. Save the mustard greens for a dinner
that needs some spicing up. This one doesn't.*

YIELD: 4 SERVINGS
4 boneless, skinless chicken breasts
Salt and pepper to taste
2 tablespoons butter (no substitutions)
$\frac{1}{2}$ cup dry white wine
$\frac{1}{2}$ cup crème fraîche (heavy cream—no substitutions)
3 teaspoons mustard
I cup slivered mushrooms

1. Wash the chicken pieces and pat dry. Lightly salt and pepper both sides.

2. Melt the butter in a skillet. When the butter sizzles, add the chicken pieces, and brown lightly on both sides.

3. Deglaze the pan by adding the wine, scraping to incorporate any drippings. Add the slivered mushrooms, and allow the mushrooms and chicken to simmer in the wine for 10 to 15 minutes or until the chicken is fork-tender, turning as needed. Remove the chicken to a warm platter.

4. Whisk the mustard into the cream and add to the skillet, whisking to incorporate the ingredients.

5. Bring the sauce to a simmer. Pour over the chicken, and serve.

Chicken Dijon

Chicken Dijon is the quintessential mustard dish. This low-fat, reduced-calorie recipe is an update of the classic dish that should please the health-conscious among us. Don't worry. The distinctive taste and delicious flavor remains intact. I don't like to confuse the taste buds of my guests by serving too many richly flavored dishes at the same time. Wild rice or white rice and steamed green beans (lightly cooked, slightly crunchy, and sprinkled with toasted almond slivers) or steamed broccoli are perfect with Chicken Dijon. If you want to impress a guest, serve with Savory Stuffed Orange Cups (see page 186) on the side.

YIELD: 4 SERVINGS

4 skinless boneless chicken breasts

Olive oil cooking spray

2 crushed garlic cloves (optional)

$\frac{1}{2}$ teaspoon dried tarragon

Cracked pepper to taste

Canola oil cooking spray

$\frac{3}{4}$ cup reduced-fat chicken broth, or 1 teaspoon Better Than Bouillon Chicken Base* dissolved in $\frac{3}{4}$ cup hot water

2 tablespoons Dijon-Style Mustard (see page 107)

1 teaspoon honey

$\frac{3}{4}$ cup nonfat sour cream

*Better Than Bouillon is an all-natural low-fat, low-sodium product that can add rich chicken or beef flavor to any dish. If you haven't discovered this product yet, look for it next to the bouillon cubes in most supermarkets. I recommend it.

1. Wash the chicken pieces and pat them dry. Lightly spray each piece with olive oil cooking spray.

2. If using garlic, spread a bit over each breast. Sprinkle the chicken breasts with tarragon and pepper.

3. Lightly coat a frying pan with canola oil cooking spray. Preheat the pan over medium heat.

4. When the pan is hot, add the chicken pieces. Cook for about 3 minutes on each side, or until the pieces are nicely browned. Remove the chicken pieces and set aside.

5. Reduce the heat to low and add the broth or dissolved chicken base, scraping loose any brown bits. Add the mustard and honey, and whisk well to combine.

6. Return the chicken to the pan, turning once to coat each piece. Cover, and poach the chicken in the simmering liquid for 15 or 20 minutes, turning once, or until the chicken is fork-tender and the meat is no longer pink. Remove the chicken pieces to a warm platter.

7. Whisk the sour cream into the sauce. Return the chicken to the pan to reheat, spooning sauce over each piece. Serve immediately.

Mustard-Teriyaki Chicken

This dish tastes wonderful with wild rice and a lightly dressed salad of mixed greens.

YIELD: 4 SERVINGS

4 chicken pieces (breasts and thighs)

$1/2$ cup honey mustard

3 tablespoons teriyaki sauce

1. Wash the chicken and pat dry. Set aside.

2. Combine the mustard and teriyaki sauce. Reserve $1/3$ cup of this sauce.

3. Put the chicken pieces in the remaining sauce, turning to coat. Refrigerate for 2 hours.

4. Grill or broil the chicken 4 to 6 inches from the heat source until fork-tender—about ten minutes per side. Brush the pieces with the reserved sauce frequently.

Mustard Chicken and Souper Rice

If I remember correctly, this recipe dates back to the 1950s, but it may have been around longer than that. This chicken and rice dish has gone through countless variations, I'm sure, as cooks all over the world added their own touches. This recipe uses the soup can as a measuring device. To make this dish most appealing to the eye, it should be accompanied by something green. Steamed mustard greens, spinach, or broccoli are all wonderful choices. If you want to add something special, add a stuffed orange cup to each plate (see page 186).

YIELD: 4 SERVINGS

4–6 pieces of boneless, skinless chicken
(breasts and thighs work best)

1 tablespoon of your favorite prepared mustard

1 $10\frac{3}{4}$-ounce can reduced-fat condensed cream of chicken soup

1 $10\frac{3}{4}$-ounce can reduced-fat condensed cream of mushroom soup

1 measuring can uncooked white rice

1 measuring can dry white wine*

*Even though the alcohol will cook away, some people may be concerned about cooking with wine. If so, select a nonalcoholic wine. You can also substitute one can of water for the wine, but you'll lose a lot of flavor.

1. Preheat the oven to 350°F.

2. Wash the chicken pieces and remove visible fat from them. Pat them dry. Spread each piece with a thin coating of prepared mustard. Set aside.

3. Pour both cans of soup into an 8-x-8 or 9-x-9 baking dish. Stir to combine.

4. Fill an empty soup can with the uncooked rice and add it to the soup. Stir to mix.

5. Fill an empty soup can with the wine. Mix the wine into the rice and soup mixture.

6. Put the prepared chicken pieces on top of the rice mixture, and cover with foil.

7. Bake the dish for 45 minutes, then remove it from the oven and take off the foil. Using a slender spoon, try to stir the rice a bit without disturbing the chicken.

8. Return uncovered to the oven and continue baking for another 45 minutes. Serve immediately.

Chicken en Papillote

"En papillote" is a favorite French method of cooking. In this style of cooking, the ingredients are wrapped in parchment paper and baked. Foil isn't as elegant, but it works equally well. Perhaps I should have called this recipe "Chicken en Foil Américaine." What do you think? Wild rice and honey-mustard-glazed carrots ensure a pretty presentation, and they taste wonderful with the chicken. I must have something green at every meal. If you feel the same way, add a green salad.

YIELD: 4 SERVINGS

4 boneless, skinless chicken breasts or thighs
2 egg yolks
2 tablespoons mustard
1 tablespoon olive oil
$\frac{1}{4}$ cup celery, very finely minced
1 teaspoon dried tarragon, crumbled
Salt and pepper to taste
4 10-inch squares of aluminum foil

1. Preheat the oven to 350°F.

2. Wash the chicken and pat dry. Set aside.

3. Beat the egg yolks and whisk in the mustard and oil. Coat the chicken pieces with this mixture.

4. Put each piece of chicken on one square of foil. Sprinkle each piece with the minced celery, tarragon, and salt and pepper.

5. Close the foil securely around the chicken. Bake it for 30 minutes, or until the chicken is fork-tender.

Bourbon Beef With Mustard Sauce

This is a very rich dish. Serve with boiled potatoes dressed with a bit of butter and parsley, or plain white rice. Steamed broccoli is the perfect accompaniment.

YIELD: 4 SERVINGS
3 cups water
2 pounds round steak
I medium onion, coarsely chopped
2 cloves garlic, quartered
2 bay leaves
I teaspoon salt
I tablespoon olive oil
2 cups beef broth
$\frac{1}{2}$ cup bourbon
I tablespoon Dijon-Style Mustard (see page 107 for recipe)
2 teaspoons flour
2 tablespoons sour cream

1. Combine water, steak, onion, garlic, bay leaves, and salt in a heavy pan. Cover, and cook over medium-high heat for about 45 minutes, or until the water evaporates.

2. Reduce the heat to medium. Add the olive oil, and brown the meat on both sides.

3. Add the beef broth and bourbon. Cover the pan and cook for 20 to 30 minutes, or until the liquid is reduced by half and the meat is fork-tender.

4. Remove the meat to a warm platter, and reduce the heat under the sauce to low. Slice the meat thinly.

5. In a small bowl, stir the mustard and flour into the sour cream. Add this mixture to the liquid remaining in the pan, stirring constantly. When the sauce is thick, about 10 to 15 minutes, pour over the sliced beef. Serve immediately.

Rabbit Saddle With Mustard Sauce

Several of the recipes in this book came directly to me from an acquaintance in France. This classic French dish is one of them. The French serve steamed spinach with this dish. I prefer mustard greens. You decide which you prefer.

YIELD: 4 SERVINGS
4 deboned rabbit saddles
2 tablespoons canola oil
2 tablespoons dried thyme
⅓ cup chicken stock
3 ounces *fromage blanc* (smooth cottage cheese)
I tablespoon mustard
2 teaspoons dried tarragon
Salt and pepper to taste

1. Preheat the oven to 325°F.

2. To prepare the saddles, oil them liberally, then sprinkle the underside of each with thyme. Tuck the edges under and shape them to look like small roasts. Tie each with string.

3. Bake the saddles for 30 to 40 minutes. Rabbit is a dry meat, so baste with the pan drippings frequently. When the saddles are done, remove to a warm plate.

4. Prepare the sauce by simmering the chicken stock until it is reduced by half. Add the pan drippings to the reduced stock. Stir in the cottage cheese, mustard, and tarragon, and whisk well until the sauce is smooth. Add salt and pepper, if needed.

5. Pour the mustard sauce on the rabbit, and serve immediately.

Fish Entrées

Mustard isn't just for meat, it also does a lot for fish. Many people shy away from fish, even though they know it's a healthy food, either because they think it's too bland or because they think it's too much trouble to fix. This section will change your mind on both counts.

Crab Salad in Tomato Cups

These crab-filled tomato cups are a nice prelude to an elegant dinner, and they also work well on a buffet. You might also use them as the centerpiece of a luncheon. The Quick Fiesta Cornbread (see page 196) makes a good accompaniment.

YIELD: 4 SERVINGS

4 medium tomatoes

8 ounces cooked crabmeat (or imitation crabmeat)

I green onion with top, finely chopped

$\frac{1}{2}$ cup celery, finely chopped

DRESSING

$\frac{1}{4}$ cup nonfat mayonnaise

I tablespoon lemon juice

$\frac{1}{4}$ teaspoon dry mustard powder

1. Prepare the cups by cutting the tops off the tomatoes in a saw-tooth pattern. Squeeze to remove seeds, and scoop out the soft pulp, leaving the sides intact. Drain out the juice and set aside.

2. To prepare the dressing, whisk the ingredients together until smooth.

3. Combine the crabmeat, onion, and celery, and toss gently to mix. Drizzle with the dressing, and toss again.

4. Fill the tomato cups generously with the salad mixture, and nest them in lettuce cups.

Smoked Salmon Salad and Napa Valley Mustard Greens With Lemon Shallot Vinaigrette

This delicious dish is one of the original mustard recipes introduced at the Napa Valley Mustard Festival in 1998. Credit goes to Andrew Sutton, Executive Chef of Auberge du Soleil.

YIELD: 8 SERVINGS

8 thin slices of smoked salmon
1 pound baby mustard greens, rinsed and dried
VINAIGRETTE
$\frac{1}{2}$ cup fresh squeezed lemon juice
1 tablespoon chopped lemon zest
$\frac{1}{4}$ cup minced shallots
1 cup extra virgin olive oil
1 tablespoon honey
Salt and pepper to taste

1. To prepare the vinaigrette, put the lemon juice, zest, and shallots in a medium-sized mixing bowl, and allow to steep for 30 minutes.

2. Whisk in the olive oil and honey.

3. Season with salt and pepper.

4. Roll the salmon into 8 individual pinwheels.

5. Toss the baby mustard greens with the vinaigrette.

6. Place the greens on a plate and top with the salmon pinwheels.

Smoked Salmon Paupiettes

This is another classic French dish that came to me direct from France. It is much more elegant than the more familiar Eggs Benedict. Do try it sometime when you want to show off. My French acquaintance tells me that this entrée is often served with a chicory salad. If you want to Americanize it and serve it for a company brunch, serve these delicious little bundles on a toasted English muffin, and put some home fries on the side. Sliced tomatoes will dress up the plate and add to the appeal.

YIELD: 4 SERVINGS

¾ cup crème fraîche (heavy cream—no substitutions)
4 eggs
Water for poaching eggs
3 tablespoons vinegar
I teaspoon salt
4 slices smoked salmon
I teaspoon Dijon mustard
2 tablespoons snipped chives

1. Put the cream into a saucepan, and allow it to simmer until it is reduced by half.

2. While the cream is reducing, poach the eggs in water to which the vinegar and salt have been added.

3. Put each slice of salmon on a separate plate. Put a poached egg on top of each slice and wrap the salmon around it.

4. Complete the sauce by whisking in the mustard. Pour a little sauce over each salmon paupiette and sprinkle with the snipped chives.

Easy Salmon Patties

If the previous recipe sounds like too much trouble, try these easy and delicious patties. Dress them up with a spoonful of Rèmoulade Sauce (see page 143). My family likes these patties with broiled tomatoes and boiled potatoes sprinkled with snipped green onions.

YIELD: 4 SERVINGS

1 16-ounce can of salmon (Red Alaska Sockeye salmon is the most flavorful.)
$\frac{1}{2}$ cup crushed corn flakes or bread crumbs
2 teaspoons dried dill, crumbled
1 teaspoon dry mustard powder
1 tablespoon lemon juice
1 tablespoon melted butter (no substitutions)
1 egg (or the equivalent in egg substitute)
Salt and pepper to taste
2 tablespoons canola or olive oil

1. Drain the liquid from the can of salmon. Remove the skin and bones, and break up the salmon.

2. Combine the remaining ingredients with the salmon. Form into 4 patties (similar to hamburgers).

3. Preheat a skillet over medium heat. When the pan is hot, put in 2 tablespoons of canola or olive oil and swirl to coat the pan.

4. Cook the patties until they are lightly browned on both sides, about 7 minutes per side. Serve immediately.

Dijon-Style Trout

*My French friend who supplied this recipe says this dish should be
served with steamed potatoes. To complete the feast, add a salad
of mixed baby greens lightly dressed with Easy Honey-Mustard
Vinaigrette (see page 133), and don't forget the crusty French bread.*

YIELD: 4 SERVINGS
4 very fresh trout
5 cups court bouillon prepared according to package directions (see page 174)
SAUCE
2 shallots, chopped
I bunch parsley, chopped
$\frac{1}{4}$ cup wine vinegar
2 egg yolks
2 tablespoons Dijon-Style Mustard (see page 107)
5 tablespoons softened butter
Salt and pepper to taste

1. To prepare the sauce, in a medium-sized saucepan, simmer the
chopped shallots and parsley in the vinegar. Allow the mixture
to reduce by half. Set aside.

2. In a separate bowl, combine the egg yolks and mustard with the
softened butter. Add salt and pepper to taste.

3. Drizzle the reduced vinegar mixture into the mustard/butter
mixture. Return the sauce mixture to the saucepan and simmer,
stirring constantly, to cook the egg and thicken the sauce.

4. Bring the court bouillon to a simmer and poach the trout for 3
minutes.

5. Drain the fish and put them on a warm platter. Coat with the
mustard sauce and serve immediately.

Quick and Easy Scallops Flambé

Serve this dish with wild rice, and put something green on the plate, like mustard greens, spinach, or broccoli. Add a tangy fruit salad, if you like, and enjoy the feast.

YIELD: 4 SERVINGS
½ package instant court bouillon prepared according to package directions (see "Court Bouillon" on page 174)
1 pound scallops, fresh or frozen and thawed
2 tablespoons butter (no substitutions)
2 tablespoons prepared tarragon or dill mustard (see the recipe for Herbaceous Mustard on page 113)
¼ cup heavy cream (no substitutions)
Salt and pepper to taste
1 tablespoon cognac

1. Bring the court bouillon to a simmer over low heat. Add the scallops, and poach them for 5 minutes. Drain and set aside. Discard the poaching liquid.

2. Heat the butter in a large skillet until it bubbles around the edges. Add the drained scallops and sauté them until lightly browned on both sides—about 5 minutes.

3. Add the cognac and light a flame to it. When the flames die, remove the scallops with a slotted spoon and put them on a warm plate. Leave the liquid in the pan.

4. Pour the cream into the pan, and stir in the mustard. Taste the sauce and add salt and pepper, if needed. Simmer the sauce for 2 or 3 minutes.

5. Pour over the scallops and serve immediately.

Crusty Cod

This dish is nice with rice or macaroni and cheese and a well-dressed green salad.

4 6-ounce cod filets

2 tablespoons prepared mustard

⅓ cup bread crumbs

Canola cooking spray

1. Preheat the oven to 350°F.

2. Spread mustard thinly on one side of the filets.

3. Put the bread crumbs into a shallow dish. Press the mustard-dressed side of the filet into the bread crumbs, coating well. Do the same with the other side of the fish. The mustard not only adds nonfat flavor, but it also helps the crumbs adhere.

4. Prepare a baking sheet by spraying it lightly with canola cooking spray, then arrange the filets on it. Spray the tops of the crumbed filets lightly with canola cooking spray.

5. Bake the filets for 10 to 15 minutes, or until the fish flakes easily when tested with a fork. Don't overcook. Serve immediately.

Court Bouillon

Several of the recipes in this section call for court bouillon. Court bouillon is a rich vegetable broth used for poaching. Sometimes wine or vinegar is added. The instant variety available in your supermarket makes poaching fish easy. Court bouillon adds delicate flavor to fish, but if you can't find it, poach the fish in water to which 2 teaspoons of lemon juice have been added.

Foil-Baked Fish Filets

Select your favorite firm fish, such as sole, snapper, orange roughy, or flounder. These filets are baked in a foil pouch, which allows the fish to steam in its own juices, sealing in flavor and nutrients. The vegetables, herbs, and wine add flavor and color. A baked potato topped with nonfat sour cream and snipped green onions is the perfect accompaniment to this high-flavor, low-calorie dish.

YIELD: 4 SERVINGS
4 6-ounce fish filets
4 tablespoons dry white wine
1 tablespoon dried dill
$\frac{1}{2}$ tablespoon dry mustard powder
2 cups snow peas
2 cups very thinly slivered carrots
$\frac{1}{4}$ cup snipped green onions
Salt and pepper to taste

1. Preheat the oven to 450°F.

2. Cut heavy-duty aluminum foil into four 8-x-12-inch pieces. Center a fish filet on each piece.

3. Spoon one tablespoon of wine over each piece.

4. Combine the dill and mustard powder and sprinkle an equal amount over each filet.

5. Distribute the snow peas, slivered carrots, and snipped green onions equally over the dressed filets. Add salt and pepper to taste, if desired.

6. Bring the edges of the foil together at the top, and fold twice to seal. Don't wrap the fish too tightly. Allow space for heat circulation and expansion.

7. Arrange the pouches on a baking pan and bake for about 15 minutes, or until the thickest part of the fish flakes easily.

8. Carefully open the top seal, and serve the fish in their pouches.

Meatless Entrées and Cheese Dishes

Mustard enhances almost any dish, and cheese and mustard go together so well. The mustard adds the perfect flavor to any kind of cheese. More importantly, this pungent condiment is an essential ingredient in cheese-based dishes if you've made the switch to healthier low-fat and nonfat cheeses. Whether you're a traditionalist who insists on old-style cheese or are watching your cholesterol and counting fat grams, just use the cheese of your choice in all of the following recipes.

Hurry-up Pasta Primavera

This is pasta primavera without the fat and the fuss. You can fix this dish in the time it takes to boil the pasta. This dish is excellent with a fruit salad and crusty breadsticks.

YIELD: 4 SERVINGS

8 ounces of pasta, any shape

1 8-ounce bag of frozen mixed vegetables

1 cup nonfat sour cream

1 tablespoon of your favorite prepared mustard

1. In separate pots, boil the pasta and the vegetables according to package directions.

2. Drain the pasta and the vegetables, then combine the two in the pasta pot.

3. Stir in the sour cream and mustard.

Traditional Old-Style Quiche

This hearty and delicious dish will receive a warm welcome. In spite of that famous saying "Real men don't eat quiche," believe me, they'll gobble this one up. The men in your family will love this dish.

YIELD: 4–6 SERVINGS

1 8-inch unbaked pie shell
2 cups nonfat milk
1 cup Swiss cheese, grated
$\frac{1}{2}$ cup diced ham or bacon bits (optional)
$\frac{1}{2}$ tablespoon prepared mustard
1 teaspoon minced onion
$\frac{1}{4}$ teaspoon salt
Cracked pepper to taste
4 eggs

1. Preheat the oven to 425°F.

2. Place one unbaked pie shell in an 8-inch pie pan.

3. Heat the milk over medium-high heat until small bubbles form along the edges.

4. Reduce the heat to low and add the cheese, stirring until the cheese is melted.

5. Stir in the ham or bacon.

6. Stir in the onion, salt, and pepper, then remove from heat.

7. Beat the eggs until they are fluffy.

8. Gradually add the eggs to the cheese mixture, combining thoroughly.

9. Pour the cheese mixture into the pie shell.

10. Wrap the edges of the pastry with strips of aluminum foil to protect the crust from browning too quickly.

11. Bake the quiche for 10 minutes.

12. Reduce the heat to 325°F and continue baking for 20 to 30 minutes, or until a toothpick inserted in the center comes out clean.

Crustless Low-Cal Quiche

A lightly dressed hearty salad of mixed greens tossed with slivers of green, red, and yellow peppers; thinly sliced red onions; and chunks of ripe tomato complement either of these flavorful quiches. Refrigerate leftovers promptly. If you're lucky enough to have a serving or two left, enjoy it cold the next day for lunch.

YIELD: 4–6 SERVINGS

4 eggs or the equivalent in egg substitute
$\frac{1}{4}$ cup flour
$\frac{1}{2}$ teaspoon baking powder
$\frac{1}{4}$ teaspoon salt
$\frac{1}{2}$ tablespoon prepared mustard
$\frac{1}{4}$ cup minced onion
I cup nonfat milk
I cup broccoli florets, slivered; or I cup cooked spinach, drained and chopped
2 cups nonfat cottage cheese
2 cups of your favorite low-fat or nonfat cheese, grated
Cracked pepper to taste

1. Preheat the oven to 425°F.

2. In a large bowl, beat the eggs until they are fluffy.

3. Sift in the flour, baking powder, and salt, and beat until well combined.

4. Stir in the mustard and milk. Add broccoli or spinach and combine.

5. Add cheeses and stir thoroughly.

6. Spray a 9-inch pie plate with canola cooking spray, and pour the cheese mixture into the prepared pan.

7. Bake for 10 minutes.

8. Reduce heat to 350°F and continue baking for 20 to 30 minutes, or until a toothpick inserted in the center comes out clean. Slice and serve immediately.

Eggplant Casserole

This hearty eggplant casserole is good enough to serve as the star of the show if your family likes eggplant. You can also rely on it when you're serving leftovers and need to round the meal out with something substantial.

YIELD: 4 SERVINGS

1–2 tablespoons olive oil

½ cup diced onion

1 garlic clove, crushed (optional)

2 medium-sized tomatoes, coarsely chopped

3 tablespoons flat-leaf parsley, snipped

½ teaspoon dry mustard powder

Salt and cracked pepper to taste

2 medium eggplants, peeled and thinly sliced

1. Preheat the oven to 350°F.

2. Lightly sauté the onion and garlic in the olive oil. Stir in the tomatoes and parsley and sprinkle with mustard powder, adding salt and pepper to taste. Set aside.

3. Grease a medium-sized baking dish liberally with olive oil. Alternate layers of eggplant slices and sauce, beginning with the eggplant and finishing with sauce on the top.

4. Bake for about 40 minutes, or until the eggplant is fork tender. If you wish, sprinkle a little grated cheese on top. Serve immediately.

Family Fondue

You don't need a fondue pot with this easy recipe. Select a heavy pot, preferably one with two small handles, and cook the fondue on your stove. Fondue is a wonderful choice for a gathering of guests, and it can be the basis for a fun family meal. This recipe is ample for four hearty eaters. It can be doubled (or even quadrupled) if you're serving a crowd.

YIELD: 4 SERVINGS
I cup dry white wine
I tablespoon cornstarch
I clove garlic, peeled and halved
I ½ teaspoon lemon juice
12 ounces cheese of your choice, grated*
I teaspoon of your favorite mustard (Dijon or tarragon mustard are both excellent choices)
¼ teaspoon Worcestershire sauce
Pinch of garlic powder (optional)
3 drops Tabasco sauce (optional)

* For a traditional fondue, use 6 ounces grated Gruyère cheese and 6 ounces grated Emmenthaler or Jarlsberg cheese. For a heartier American-style fondue, substitute 6 ounces of grated sharp Cheddar cheese for one of those more traditional soft white cheeses. To reduce calories and fat grams, select low-fat or nonfat cheeses.

1. Combine cornstarch and one tablespoon of the wine in a small bowl and set aside.

2. Rub the insides of a small pot with both halves of the garlic clove.

3. Add the remaining wine to the garlic-perfumed pot, and heat over medium-high heat on the stove. When the wine is hot but not boiling, add the lemon juice.

4. Turn the heat very low and slowly add the cheeses, stirring constantly. Continue cooking and stirring until the fondue is smooth.

5. Add the mustard, Worcestershire sauce, garlic, and Tabasco sauce.

6. When thoroughly blended, add the cornstarch and wine mixture and stir until the fondue bubbles and thickens.

If you're using a fondue pot, transfer the fondue to the pot, or just leave the finished fondue in its cooking pot and put it in the middle of the table. Keep it warm over a candle flame or can of Sterno. Long-handled fondue forks for dipping are nice but not really necessary. Regular dinner forks will do. Provide torn chunks of French and sourdough bread, wedges of apple, and stalks of celery for dipping. A big bowl of tossed greens, thinly sliced onions, green peppers, and juicy tomatoes tossed with a light vinaigrette dressing will complement the meal perfectly. A selection of antipasto favorites, such as ham, salami, and roast beef, are also good for dipping. Select low-fat varieties of the meats, and enjoy with a clear conscience. To complete the feast, be sure to set out a selection of hearty mustards.

Rich Tomato Rarebit

Try serving this or any of these rarebits hot over broiled tomatoes.
(See the recipe for Broiled Tomatoes on page 197).
A lightly dressed salad of mixed greens or juicy fruit rounds out this
nearly forgotten feast perfectly. For a heartier meal, accompany
it with one of the bean salads in the "Hearty Salads" section.

YIELD: 4–6 SERVINGS
I can condensed tomato soup
I cup (8 ounces) sharp cheese, grated
I teaspoon of your favorite prepared mustard
I teaspoon Worcestershire sauce
1/8 teaspoon salt
2 eggs or the equivalent in egg substitute

1. In a heavy saucepan, heat the soup over very low heat.

2. When the soup is hot, add the cheese. Stir constantly until the cheese is melted and the mixture is smooth. Remove from heat.

3. Add the mustard, Worcestershire sauce, and salt. Stir to combine.

4. Beat the eggs until they are fluffy, and stir into the mixture.

5. Cook over very low heat, stirring constantly until the rarebit is hot.

Welsh Rarebit With Beer

*Welsh rarebit is a delicious, somewhat old-fashioned cheese dish served
hot over toast or crackers. My grandmother was famous for her rich
Welsh rarebit, and served it often at her "lady's luncheons."
My mother favored it for Sunday night supper, and she
often used up odds and ends of cheese, depending on
what was in the kitchen at the time. The more
flavorful the cheese, the better the dish.
Low-fat or nonfat cheese may be used.*

YIELD: 4–6 SERVINGS

1 tablespoon butter (no substitutions)
1 cup beer
2 cups (16 ounces) sharp cheese, grated
1 egg
$\frac{1}{2}$ teaspoon prepared mustard
1 teaspoon Worcestershire sauce
1 teaspoon salt
$\frac{1}{2}$ teaspoon paprika
$\frac{1}{4}$ teaspoon curry powder (optional)

1. Melt the butter in a double boiler over (not in) boiling water. Stir in the beer.

2. When the mixture is warm, add the cheese. Stir constantly until the cheese is melted.

3. Whisk the egg until it is frothy, and stir it into the cheese mixture.

4. Add the spices and seasonings. Continue stirring until the rarebit is very hot and the sauce is perfectly smooth.

5. Serve hot over toast or crisp crackers.

Welsh Rarebit With Milk

The original recipe for this rarebit called for heavy cream, but we know better than to use that today. If you're really counting fat grams, use low-fat or nonfat milk.

YIELD: 4–6 SERVINGS

I tablespoon butter (no substitutions)
2 cups (16 ounces) sharp cheese of your choice, grated
$\frac{1}{2}$ teaspoon prepared mustard
I teaspoon Worcestershire sauce
I teaspoon salt
$\frac{1}{2}$ teaspoon paprika
$\frac{1}{4}$ teaspoon curry powder (optional)
$\frac{3}{4}$–I cup milk

1. Melt the butter in a double boiler over (not in) boiling water. Add the cheese, and stir until the cheese is melted.

2. Stir in the seasonings.

3. Heat the milk.

4. Slowly stir the milk into the cheese mixture, blending thoroughly. Add the hot milk until the rarebit is a good consistency. You may not need the full cup.

5. Continue stirring until the rarebit is very hot and the sauce is perfectly smooth.

Macaroni & Cheese

All you really need with this dish is a well-dressed salad of mixed greens, but some pickled beets (see page 155) on the side make a pretty picture, and they taste great, too.

YIELD: 4 SERVINGS
8 ounces macaroni, any style
1 clove garlic, halved
½ cup nonfat milk
1 egg yolk, beaten
4 tablespoons butter (no substitutions)
4 ounces cheese, grated
2 tablespoons prepared mustard
Salt and pepper to taste

1. Cook the macaroni as directed on the package. Drain and set aside.

2. Rub all sides of an 8-x-8- or 9-x-9-inch ovenproof dish or pan with the cut sides of the garlic clove.

3. In a saucepan, whisk the beaten egg yolk into the milk. Heat to simmering, then whisk in the remaining ingredients. Allow the sauce to simmer until the cheese is melted and the sauce has thickened a little.

4. Combine the sauce with the drained macaroni and pour into the prepared pan. Bake at 350°F for 20 to 25 minutes, or until the dish is bubbling and the top is lightly browned.

Interesting Side Dishes and Breads

An interesting side dish may be just what you need to perk up a quick family meal, or to dress up a dinner party. Check out these recipes.

Fried Rice With Cucumber

This recipe from India is a nice change from ordinary steamed rice.
It is both flavorful and refreshing all at once.
I think you'll enjoy it.

YIELD: 4 SERVINGS

1 tablespoon mustard oil
$\frac{1}{2}$ teaspoon mustard seeds
1 cup sweet onion, thinly sliced
1 cup cucumber, finely diced
4 cups cooked rice
$\frac{1}{2}$ teaspoon salt

1. Heat the oil in a wok or skillet.

2. Add the mustard seeds and onion. Cook, stirring until the onion is tender—about 5 minutes.

3. Add the cucumber, and stir until the cucumber is heated through.

4. Add the cooked rice, sprinkle on salt, and toss with other ingredients. Cook, stirring frequently, until the rice is hot. Serve immediately.

Savory Stuffed Orange Cups

This surprising delight is the perfect complement to almost any meal.

YIELD: 4 SERVINGS

2 cups herb-seasoned cubed stuffing
$1/2$ teaspoon dry mustard powder
I tablespoon butter (no substitutions)
$1/4$ teaspoon poultry seasoning
$1/3$ cup chopped onion
$1/3$ cup chopped celery
$1/3$ cup chicken broth, or I teaspoon Better Than Bouillon* dissolved in $1/3$ cup water
2 large oranges

*Better Than Bouillon is an all-natural low-fat, low-sodium product that can add rich chicken or beef flavor to any dish. If you haven't discovered this product yet, look for it next to the bouillon cubes in most supermarkets. I recommend it.

1. Preheat the oven to 350°F.

2. Put the seasoned bread cubes into a medium-sized bowl and sprinkle with mustard powder and poultry seasoning.

3. Melt the butter in a saucepan. Add the chopped onion and celery and sauté lightly.

4. Stir in the chicken broth, and let the vegetables simmer over very low heat.

5. Cut the oranges in half. Scoop out the meat of the orange, catching the juice in a measuring cup. Reserve the orange sections, and put the orange cups to one side.

6. Cut the orange sections into pieces and put them in the measuring cup with the juice. You should end up with about a $3/4$ cup of juice and orange pieces, but the measurement is not critical. Just use what you end up with.

7. Drizzle the vegetables and broth over the bread cubes, mustard powder, and poultry seasoning, and toss well to mix. Add the orange juice and pieces and combine.

8. Pack one-fourth of the stuffing mixture into each orange cup. Arrange the stuffed oranges in a baking dish and cover with foil.

9. Bake for 20 minutes. Remove the foil and cook for 10 minutes longer.

10. Serve hot.

Celeriac in Mustard Sauce

Celeriac (celery root) is an excellent change from the usual vegetables. Because of the way it is prepared in this recipe, the characteristic bitterness of celeriac is lessened.

YIELD: 2–4 SERVINGS
1 large celery root (about 1 pound)
1 ½ teaspoons lemon juice
3 tablespoons of your favorite prepared mustard
3 tablespoons hot water
2 tablespoons apple cider vinegar
6 tablespoons olive oil
½ teaspoon tarragon, dried
Salt and cracked pepper to taste
4 tablespoons chopped parsley
4 tablespoons capers (optional)

1. Scrub the root, peel it, and cut it into matchsticks. Drop the celeriac in a pot of boiling water to which the lemon juice has been added. Blanch for 2 minutes. Drain and cool.

2. In a blender, combine the mustard, hot water, and vinegar. While blending, drizzle in the oil. Adding the oil slowly will prevent the mixture from separating. When the dressing is nicely thickened, add the tarragon, salt, and pepper.

3. Pour the dressing over the blanched celeriac and allow it to marinate for 2 to 3 hours at room temperature.

4. Just before serving, sprinkle with parsley and capers. Serve at room temperature.

Okra and Potatoes

Because it calls for sautéed mustard seeds, cumin, and curry,
this recipe has a decidedly Middle Eastern flavor.

YIELD: 4 SERVINGS
4 medium unpeeled potatoes, scrubbed and diced
2 cups okra, washed, trimmed, and diced
6 tablespoons canola oil, divided
I teaspoon mustard seeds
I teaspoon cumin seeds
I teaspoon curry powder
$\frac{1}{2}$ teaspoon turmeric
$\frac{1}{2}$ teaspoon cayenne (optional)
Salt and cracked pepper to taste

1. Heat a frying pan over medium heat. Coat the pan with 3 tablespoons of oil. Brown the potatoes in the hot oil, and cook until tender.

2. Drop the diced okra into a saucepan of boiling water. Cover and simmer until the okra is tender, about 5 to 8 minutes. Drain well.

3. Heat the remaining 3 tablespoons of oil in a large frying pan just until it begins to smoke. Add the mustard seeds to the hot oil. Stir until they begin to pop. If the oil splatters, top the pan with a lid and shake it (as if you were popping popcorn) until the seeds pop. Add the cumin seeds, and brown lightly. Add the other spices, stirring constantly. Turn off the heat.

4. Add the browned potatoes and cooked okra to the pan. Toss the vegetables with the spices and combine well. Serve immediately.

Indian Eggplant

This eggplant calls for "panch phoron," a spicy blend of the spices of India that includes mustard seed, kalonji, fennel, fenugreek, and cumin. This is a beautiful mix of the whole seeds. It is intensely flavorful and spicy but milder than you would expect. Panch phoron can be found at Indian markets.

YIELD: 4 SERVINGS
2 tablespoons mustard or canola oil
I cup thinly sliced sweet onion
2 teaspoons ginger root, slivered
I green chili, diced (optional)
I teaspoon panch phoron
I teaspoon coriander
I teaspoon sugar
2 small eggplants, washed and cut into bite-sized chunks
I teaspoon salt
I teaspoon dry chili powder
$3/4$ cup warm water

1. In a wok or skillet, heat the oil. Add the onion, ginger, and diced chili, and cook until the onion is tender, about 3 to 4 minutes.

2. Add the panch phoron, coriander, and sugar. Stir to combine.

3. Add the eggplant chunks, salt, chili powder, and water, stirring to combine. Cook until the eggplant is tender, about 8 to 10 minutes. Serve immediately over rice.

French-Style Mushrooms

My French friend suggests serving these mushrooms with a
spinach salad and rice pilaf. Sounds good to me.

YIELD: 4 SERVINGS
3 pounds fresh mushrooms, cleaned and cut into thick slices
Juice of two lemons
4 tablespoons butter
2 shallots
½ cup heavy cream
I egg yolk
2 tablespoons Dijon-style prepared mustard (see page 107)
½ cup dry white wine
Salt and white pepper to taste
2 green onions, minced

1. Put the juice of one lemon and half the butter in a medium-sized saucepan. Heat over low heat until the butter melts.

2. Add the mushrooms. Cover and simmer until the juices are drawn out.

3. Drain the mushrooms, reserving broth. Simmer the broth over low heat until it is reduced by half, and set aside.

4. Sauté the shallots in the remaining butter over low heat. Add the mushrooms to the shallots, and simmer for 10 minutes over low heat.

5. In a small bowl, whisk the cream and egg yolk together. Add the mustard, white wine, broth reduction, and juice of the remaining lemon. Add salt and white pepper to taste. Simmer until the egg is cooked and the sauce is thickened.

6. Add the mushrooms, and toss to coat with the sauce. Simmer until the mushrooms are heated through.

7. Sprinkle with chopped green onions and serve immediately.

Spicy Canned Baked Beans

Some canned baked beans are well flavored, but most are way too "soupy." The obvious way around that is to discard most of the liquid. Here's how to make canned baked beans taste like homemade.

Yield: 10–12 servings
1 27-ounce can baked beans
$\frac{1}{4}$ cup onion, finely chopped
$\frac{1}{8}$ cup green pepper, finely chopped
$\frac{1}{8}$ cup celery, finely chopped
2 tablespoons olive oil
4 tablespoons ketchup
2 tablespoons dark molasses or brown sugar
$\frac{1}{2}$ tablespoon dry mustard

1. Preheat the oven to 375°F.

2. Open the beans and drain them, reserving the juice: Open the can, leaving the lid in place. Then tip the can and drain the juice into a cup.

3. Sauté the onions, green pepper, and celery lightly in the olive oil. Do not permit them to brown.

4. Add the sautéed vegetables along with the ketchup, molasses, and mustard to the drained beans, tossing lightly to combine. If the mixture is too dry, add a little of the reserved bean juice.

5. Place the mixture in a baking dish that has been treated with canola oil cooking spray. Cover with foil. Bake the beans for 30 minutes.

6. Remove the cover for about the last 10 minutes of cooking time to allow the beans to develop a delicious top crust.

Variation: If you don't want to turn on the oven, or if you're in a hurry, you can cook these spicy "dressed-up" beans on the stovetop. Make sure they bubble merrily for at least 10 minutes to meld flavors. Stir often to prevent sticking.

Old-Style Baked Beans

These are the kind of beans grandma used to make.

YIELD: 4 SERVINGS
1 ½ cups dried beans (navy or white)
¼ cup diced onion
3 tablespoons dark molasses
3 tablespoons ketchup
1 tablespoon dry mustard
1 teaspoon salt
3 slices smoked turkey bacon

1. Preheat the oven to 250°F.

2. Prepare the beans according to package directions. When the beans are cooked, drain them, saving the cooking liquid.

3. Add the diced onion, molasses, ketchup, mustard powder, and salt to the cooked beans, tossing to combine. Drizzle 1/4 cup of the reserved liquid over the beans. Place them in a baking dish that has been treated with canola oil cooking spray. Arrange the bacon on top of the beans, and cover with foil.

4. Bake the dish at 250°F for 6 to 8 hours. Check on the beans, and stir them occasionally. If they become too dry, add a little of the reserved cooking liquid.

5. Remove the cover for the last 30 minutes of cooking time to allow the bacon to crisp and the beans to develop a delicious top crust.

Mustard-Seed Biscuits

*I can't think of any meal, including breakfast, where these and
the following Quick-Fix Mustard-Seed Drop Biscuits
would not be welcomed. I like my biscuits drizzled
with honey. These are no exception.*

YIELD: 14 BISCUITS

2 cups all-purpose flour
1 tablespoon baking powder
$1/4$ teaspoon salt
1 tablespoon mustard seeds
5 tablespoons cold butter, cut into small pieces
1 cup buttermilk
1 tablespoon spicy brown mustard
Canola oil cooking spray
1 egg or the equivalent in egg substitute

1. Preheat the oven to 400°F.

2. Mix together the flour, baking powder, salt, and mustard seeds.

3. Add the butter. Pulse in a food processor (or cut in with a pastry blender) until the mixture resembles coarse meal.

4. Add buttermilk and mustard. Mix just until the ingredients come together. The mixture will be very moist.

5. Knead the dough on a floured board until it holds together and is smooth. Add a little extra flour to keep it from sticking, if necessary. Use a light hand and don't overknead.

6. Roll the dough into a $1/2$-inch-thick log. Cut into rounds, reusing scraps as needed.

7. Spritz a cookie sheet with canola oil cooking spray. Place the biscuits about one inch apart on the greased sheet.

8. Mix the egg with a fork until frothy. Brush on biscuits.

9. Bake the biscuits until golden, about 15 minutes. Serve hot from the oven.

Mustard Greens

There are many ways to enjoy mustard greens. Mustard greens are almost as important as collard greens in old-style Southern cooking, and they're a staple in parts of Asia. The greens are high in vitamins, especially vitamins A, B, and C. It's been reported that a daily serving of mustard greens will cure scurvy, a disease caused by a lack of vitamin C. If you don't have mustard greens growing in your garden, you'll need to purchase about one bunch for two servings. Some supermarkets carry mustard greens, some do not. However, your local farmer's market, co-op, or organic produce market will usually offer them.

Mustard greens, especially mature leaves, have a bitter taste. This is a characteristic of the plant that I enjoy, probably because it's a "comfort food" from my past. However, if you find the leaves too bitter for your palate, twice-cooking solves the problem: Cook the leaves in boiling salted water to cover for 5 minutes, then drain and discard the water. Much of the bitterness will drain away with the cooking liquid. Cook the greens again by any method.

Once you get acquainted, you may find that these spicy leaves have become a favorite in your house. Incorporating mustard greens into your meals is easy. Here are a few ideas to get you started.

1. The frilly leaves of the mustard plant—either alone or in combination with other greens—are terrific in salads. Simply wash the leaves, remove the heavy center rib, tear the fronds, and toss them into a salad bowl. Dress lightly so as not to overwhelm their distinctive flavor.

2. When stir-frying vegetables (in a scant tablespoon of olive or canola oil), add torn mustard greens when the other vegetables are tender. Cook another 30 seconds or so. Serve immediately.

3. For an extra dose of flavor, add chopped mustard greens to soups and stews.

4. Steamed greens are a favorite in my house. Like all greens, mustard greens cook down as they wilt. Prepare the greens by washing them well and removing the heavy center rib, then steam them until tender, about 5 to 10 minutes. Serve with vinegar or lemon juice, if you wish.

5. If you don't have a steamer, you can still steam the leaves if you're careful. Prepare the greens by washing them well and removing the heavy center rib. Leave them wet and dripping. Put them into a heavy pot and cover. Over a low fire, cook the greens for about six minutes, or until tender. The water clinging to the leaves will provide the steam.

Quick-Fix Mustard-Seed Drop Biscuits

If you are in a hurry, these quick mustard-seed biscuits are a fine replacement for the original.

YIELD: 12 BISCUITS

2 $\frac{1}{4}$ cups baking mix

1 tablespoon mustard seeds

1 tablespoon prepared mustard

$\frac{2}{3}$ cup milk

1. Preheat the oven to 450°F.

2. Combine baking mix and mustard seeds.

3. Add the milk and mustard and stir until a soft dough forms.

4. Drop the dough by tablespoonsful onto an ungreased cookie sheet.

5. Bake for 8 to 10 minutes, or until the top peaks are golden brown. Serve immediately.

Variation: If you wish, you may knead the dough, roll it into a $\frac{1}{2}$-inch-thick log, cut out the biscuits, and bake as directed in the recipe for Mustard-Seed Biscuits on page 193. If you're in a hurry, don't bother. Drop biscuits aren't as pretty as rolled biscuits, but they are just as tasty.

Quick Fiesta Cornbread

Fiesta Cornbread is a spicy treat. Steamed mustard greens drizzled with vinegar and chunks of this cornbread hot from the oven are a favorite quick meal in my house, but don't be afraid to serve it to guests (with Fricassee of Chicken With Black-Eyed Peas, perhaps, see page 160), or use it to deliciously round out a skimpy family meal. It's good cold the next day, too.

YIELD: 6 SERVINGS
1 box prepared cornbread mix
Nonfat sour cream
Mustard (dry or prepared)
Salsa

1. Prepare the cornbread according to the manufacturer's instructions; however, use nonfat sour cream in place of the milk called for in the package instructions, and for every cup of dry mix, stir into the prepared batter: $1/2$ teaspoon dry mustard powder, or 1 teaspoon prepared mustard; and $1/3$ cup chunky salsa

2. Bake according to the manufacturer's directions, or until a toothpick inserted in the center comes out clean. This is a heavy, moist batter; it may take a little longer to bake.

Broiled Tomatoes

Broiled tomatoes are wonderful with any cheese dish,
and they can also dress up any dinner plate.

YIELD: 4 SERVINGS

2 medium tomatoes

$\frac{1}{4}$ cup nonfat mayonnaise

1 tablespoon minced parsley

1 $\frac{1}{2}$ teaspoons of your favorite mustard

$\frac{1}{4}$ teaspoon garlic or celery salt (optional)

Cracked pepper to taste

$\frac{1}{4}$ cup unseasoned prepared bread crumbs

1. Wash the tomatoes, pat them dry, and remove the stem end. Cut in half horizontally.

2. Combine the mayonnaise, parsley, mustard, salt, and pepper. Spread the sauce equally on the tomato halves.

3. Sprinkle the tomatoes with bread crumbs, and press down on them lightly.

4. Broil the tomatoes about five inches away from the heat until the tops are lightly browned and bubbly—about 5 minutes.

Warm Peach-Mustard Compote

This delicious compote was presented by Andrew Sutton, Executive Chef of Auberge du Soleil, at the Napa Valley Mustard Festival in 1998. It was warmly received. The chef likes this compote served with baked ham or grilled meats and sausages.

YIELD: 4–6 SERVINGS
I small onion, diced
2 tablespoons butter
3 ripe peaches, peeled and diced
I tablespoon maple syrup
4 ounces mild brown mustard
2 tablespoons chopped parsley
Cracked black pepper to taste

1. Sauté the onion in butter over medium heat until translucent, but not brown—approximately five minutes. Remove from heat.

2. Add the diced peaches and maple syrup. Toss gently.

3. Transfer the mixture to a medium-sized mixing bowl. Fold in the mustard, parsley, and cracked black pepper. Refrigerate for at least 4 hours.

4. Before serving, warm gently.

Bonus Recipe

Four-Star Five-Spice Gingerbread

Mustard doesn't belong in a dessert, or does it? Try this luscious gingerbread before you decide that I've completely lost my mind. It's even better the second day, and better yet the third day, if you can keep it around that long. Plan ahead—hide it.

YIELD: 10–12 SERVINGS

I cup stout or honey porter*
I cup dark (robust) molasses if you use stout, or light (mild) molasses if you use porter*
I 1/2 teaspoons baking soda
3 eggs
1/3 cup white sugar
2/3 cup dark brown sugar, packed
3/4 cup canola oil
2 cups all-purpose flour
I 1/2 teaspoons baking powder
I tablespoon ginger
I teaspoon cinnamon
1/2 teaspoon dry mustard powder
1/4 teaspoon cloves
1/4 teaspoon nutmeg

*Family and friends who sampled both the dark and light versions of this gingerbread preferred the one made with stout and dark molasses about 4 to 1. However, those who liked the lighter version said the molasses flavor apparent in the dark gingerbread was too strong for their taste. Both versions are equally rich, moist, and spicy. If your family likes molasses, by all means use stout (which is darker than porter) and dark molasses. At my house, we think an ice-cold glass of nonfat milk is the perfect accompaniment to this moist and rich gingerbread. It really needs no embellishment. If you feel you must dress it up, add a dollop of plain vanilla yogurt or dust each serving with powdered sugar.

1. Preheat the oven to 350°F.

2. Combine ale and molasses in a large saucepan. Bring to a simmer over low heat. The mixture will foam.

3. Remove from heat, and add baking soda. The mixture will foam again. Stir it down and set aside until it is cool enough to put your hand on the bottom of the pan—about 40 minutes.

4. With an electric mixer, beat the eggs and sugars together until smooth.

5. Add the oil, and beat until thoroughly combined.

6. In a separate bowl, sift the flour, baking powder, and spices together.

7. Add the liquid and dry ingredients alternately, stirring just until combined.

8. Spray a 2-inch-deep 9-x-13-inch loaf pan with canola cooking spray. Pour in the mixture and bake for 35 to 40 minutes, or until a toothpick inserted in the center comes out clean.

9. When cool, cover tightly with foil. Try to wait until the third day to serve.

Conclusion

So, now that you know all of the incredible secrets of mustard and its value in maintaining your good health, I hope you plan to increase its use in your food. Use the recipes that I have provided you with as a starting point for adding mustard to your meals. Soon you will gain a knack for adding mustard to whatever you choose. If you have mustard in your cupboard, you're ready to make something memorable. Every good cook has a "secret weapon"—a favorite ingredient he or she uses to spark up just about any dish. Good cooks taste as they cook. No matter what you happen to be making, taste as you go. If you find it needs a little something, and you just don't know what it is, try my "secret weapon"—a pinch of mustard powder or a small dab of your favorite prepared mustard—and then taste it again. Use a light hand. Even when you can't identify the pungency and bite of the mustard, you'll find it makes a difference in the taste of the dish.

I had a very good time writing this book. In fact, I enjoyed myself immensely. I hope reading it has been fun for you, as well. Now, go make some mustard!

Resources

Mustard Shops and Museums

**The Mount Horeb Mustard
Museum and Shop**
109 East Main Street
P.O. Box 468
Mount Horeb, WI 53572
Phone: (800) 438–6878
*Catalog, Newsletter, Mustards,
Pots*

**Colman's Mustard Museum
and Shop**
3 Bridewell Alley, Norwich
NR2 1AQ England
Phone: (01603) 627889
*Catalog, Mustards, Pots,
Novelty Items*

Boutique Maille
6, place de la Madeleine
Paris, France
Phone: 01 40 15 06 00
*Fresh mustards and condiments
No mail order service*

**Le Musée Amora
Boutique Moutarde Maille**
12, rue de la Liberté
Dijon, France
Phone: 03 80 30 41 02
*Fresh mustards and condiments
No mail order service*

Prepared Mustards and
Mustard Seeds, Greens, and Flours

DeGiorgi Seed Company
6011 N Street
Omaha, NE 68117
Phone: (402) 731–3901
*Catalog: Seeds; No Mustard
    Greens*

Pendery's
304 E. Belnap Street
Fort Worth, TX 76102
(800) 533–1870
*Catalog: Wild Seeds; Mustard
    Flour*

Redwood City Seed Co.
P.O. Box 361
Redwood City, CA 94064
Phone: (650) 325–7333
*Catalog: White, Black, and Brown
    Seeds; Selection of Greens*

G.B. Ratto International Grocers
821 Washington Street
Oakland, CA 94607
Phone: (510) 832–6503
*Catalog: Imported Mustards—
    Prepared and Dry*

Rafal Spice Company
2521 Russel Street
Detroit, MI 48207
Phone: (313) 259–6373
*Catalog: Black and Yellow
    Mustard Seeds*

Mustard Baths

**The Natural Therapeutics
    Centre**
Austin, TX
(512) 444–2862
Dr. Singha's Mustard Bath

Mustard Seeds

**Summers-McCann Public
    Relations**
Napa Valley Mustard Festival
110 West Napa Street
Sonoma, CA 95476
Phone: (707) 938–1133
Internet: www.winery.com/
    summers-mccann

References

Angier, Bradford. *Field Guide to Edible Wild Plants*. Harrisburg, PA: Stackpole Books, 1974.

Atlas, Ronald M. "Bioremediation." *Chemical and Engineering News.* April, 1995.

Balch, James F., M.D. and Phyllis A. Balch, C.N.C. *Prescription for Nutritional Healing*, Second Edition. Garden City Park, NY: Avery Publishing Group, 1997.

Barry, Dave. "Test Students on Subjects that Matter the Most." *The Miami Herald.* November 16, 1997.

Beale, Paul. *A Dictionary of Slang and Unconventional English*. New York: Macmillan Publishing Company, 1984.

Bernstein, Deborah, M.D. *Secrets of Fat-Free Kosher Cooking*. Garden City Park, NY: Avery Publishing Group, 1998.

Bishop, Jerry E. "Pollution Fighters Hope a Humble Weed Will Help Reclaim Contaminated Soil." *The Wall Street Journal.* August 7, 1995.

Blaylock, Michael J., et al. "Enhanced Accumulation of Pb in Indian Mustard by Soil-Applied Chelating Agents." *Environmental Science and Technology* 31(3) (1997):860–865.

Blum, H.B. and F.W. Fabian. "Spice Oils and Their Components for Controlling Microbial Surface Growth." *Fruit Products Journal* (1943).

Bremness, Lesley. *Eyewitness Handbooks: Herbs*. New York: DK Publishing, Inc., 1994.

Brown, Tom, Jr. *Tom Brown's Guide to Wild Edible and Medicinal Plants.* New York: Berkley Publishing Group, 1985.

Burlani, Arlene, R.D. *Secrets of Lactose-Free Cooking.* Garden City Park, NY: Avery Publishing Group, 1996.

Cannon, Helen L. "The Development of Botanical Methods of Prospecting for Uranium on the Colorado Plateau." *U.S. Geological Survey Bulletin 1085-A* (1960).

Carey, John. "Can Flowers Cleanse the Earth? Plants Hold Great Promise in Waste Cleanup." *Business Week* (February 19, 1996).

Carper, Jean. *The Food Pharmacy.* New York: Bantam Books, 1988.

Chin, Wee Yeow and Hsuan Keng. *Chinese Medicinal Herbs.* Sebastopol, CA: CRCS Publications, 1992.

Clarke, Charlotte Bringle. *Edible and Useful Plants of California.* Los Angeles: University of California Press, 1977.

Compestine, Ying Chang. *Secrets of Fat-Free Chinese Cooking.* Garden City Park, NY: Avery Publishing Group, 1997.

Coon, Nelson. *Using Plants for Healing.* Emmaus, PA: Rodale Press, 1979.

Dubrova, G.B., et al. "Experimental Storage of Meat in Mustard." Leningrad Soviet Trade Institute, 1951.

Dushenkov, V., et al. "Rhizofiltration: The Use of Plants to Remove Heavy Metals From Aqueous Streams." *Environmental Science and Technology* 29 (1995).

Elias, Tomas S. and Peter A. Dykeman. *Edible Wild Plants: A North American Field Guide.* New York: Sterling Publishing Co., 1990.

Flaws, Bob. *The Book of Jook: Chinese Medicinal Porridges.* Boulder, CO: Blue Poppy Press, 1995.

Flaws, Bob and H. Wolfe. *Prince Wen Hui's Cook: Chinese Dietary Therapy.* Brookline, MA: Paradigm Publications, 1983.

Frawley, David, O.M.D. *Ayurvedic Healing: A Comprehensive Guide.* Salt Lake City, UT: Passage Press, 1997.

Frawley, David O.M.D. and Dr. Vasant Lad. *The Yoga of Herbs.* Twin Lakes, WI: Lotus Press, 1992.

Futuyma, Douglas J. "The Uses of Evolutional Biology." *Science* (January 1995).

Grieve, M. *A Modern Herbal.* New York: Harcourt, Brace & Company, 1931.

Grinum, A.I. "Use of Antiseptics and Antibiotics During Storage of Carrots." Leningrad Institute, 1959.

Guyette, James E. "'Brownfields', A New Opportunity?" *Landscape Management* (October 1996).

Hasnas, Rachelle. *Bach Flower Essences.* Freedom, CA: The Crossing Press, Inc., 1997.

Heinerman, John. *Heinerman's Encyclopedia of Healing Herbs and Spices.* New York: Parker Publishing Company, 1996.

Heinerman, John. *Heinerman's Encyclopedia of Nuts, Berries and Seeds.* New York: Parker Publishing Co., Inc., 1995.

Heinerman, John. *Heinerman's New Encyclopedia of Fruits and Vegetables.* New York: Parker Publishing Company, 1995.

Hettinger, Mary E. *Home Remedies from the Bible.* New York: Globe Communications, 1996.

Howe, Peter J. "Plants Do the Dirty Work in Toxic Cleanup." *The Boston Globe* (March 10, 1997).

Hutchens, Alma R. *Indian Herbalogy of North America.* Boston, MA: Shambhala Publications, Inc., 1973.

Isaac, Susan. *Magic Hour.* New York: Harper Collins Publishers, 1991.

Jensen, Bernard. *Foods That Heal.* Garden City Park NY: Avery Publishing Group, 1988

Jensen, Ingeborg Dahl. *Wonderful,Wonderful Danish Cooking.* New York: Simon & Schuster, 1965.

Kim, Andrew H.Y. *Discover Natural Health.* Panorama City, CA: Kim's Publishing, 1988.

Kloss, Jethro. *Back to Eden. Kloss Family Heirloom Edition.* Loma Linda, CA: Back to Eden Books, 1985.

Kuman, Nanda, et al. "Phytoextraction: The Use of Plants to Remove Heavy Metals from Soils." *Environmental Science and Technology* 29 (1995).

Kumar, Amal. "Sunflowers Blossom in Tests to Remove Radioactive Metals." *The Wall Street Journal* (February 29, 1996).

Lad, Vasant. *Ayurveda: The Science of Self-Healing.* Wilmot, WI: Lotus Light, 1990.

Low, Jennie. *Chopsticks Cleaver and Wok: Homestyle Chinese Cooking.* San Francisco: Peter G. Levinson Associates, 1977.

Lu, Henry C. *Chinese Foods for Longevity.* New York: Sterling Publishing Co., Inc., 1990.

Mahoney, R.J. *When the Good Cook Gardens.* San Francisco, CA: Ortho Books, 1974.

Maoshing Ni, Ph.D. and Cathy McNease, B.S., M.H. *The Tao of Nutrition.* Santa Monica CA: SevenStar Communications, 1987.

Miller, Gustavus Hindman. *The Dictionary of Dreams.* New York: Simon & Schuster, 1992.

Muntz, Philip A. *A Flora of Southern California.* Berkeley, CA: University of California Press, 1974.

Peterson, Lee Allen. *Edible Wild Plants.* New York: Houghton Mifflin Co., 1977.

Pitchford, Paul. *Healing With Whole Foods: Oriental Traditions and Modern Nutrition.* Berkeley, CA: North Atlantic Books, 1993.

Raskin, Ilya, et al. "Removal of Radionuclide Contamination From Water by Metal-Accumulating Terrestrial Plants." Spring National Meeting: In Situ Soil and Sediment Remediation. New Orleans, 1996.

Reejhsinghni, Aroona. *Delights From Goa.* Bombay: Jaico Publishing House, 1979.

Riva, Anna. *The Modern Herbal Spellbook: The Magical Uses of Herbs.* Los Angeles: International Imports, 1993.

Riva, Anna. *Spellcraft, Hexcraft and Witchcraft.* Los Angeles: International Imports, 1990.

Robinson, L.S. and T. Corbett. *The Dreamer's Dictionary.* New York: Warner Brooks, 1974.

Spears, Richard A. *NTC's Dictionary of American Slang and Colloquial Expressions.* Lincolnwood, IL: National Textbook Company, 1989.

Tenney, Louise. *Today's Herbal Health.* Provo, UT: Woodland Books, 1983.

Tull, Delena. *A Practical Guide to Edible and Useful Plants.* Austin, TX: Texas Monthly Press, Inc., 1987.

Warrier, Gopi and Deepika Gunawant, M.D. *The Complete Illustrated Guide to Ayurveda: The Ancient Indian Healing Tradition.* Great Britain: Element Books Limited, 1997.

Weiner, M.A. *Earth Medicine/Earth Food.* New York: Ballantine Books, 1980.

Woodruff, Sandra, R.D. *Brand Name Fat-Fighter's Cookbook.* Garden City Park, NY: Avery Publishing Group, 1995.

Woodruff, Sandra, R.D. *Secrets of Fat-Free Cooking.* Garden City Park, NY: Avery Publishing Group, 1995.

Wright, David. *Diet for the 21st Century.* Vancouver, Canada: Govinda's Press, 1992.

Yee, Rhoda. *Chinese Village Cookbook.* San Francisco: Yerba Buena Press, 1975.

Zand, Janet, et al. *Smart Medicine for a Healthier Child.* Garden City Park, NY: Avery Publishing Group, 1994.

Index

Healthy Habits

are easy to come by—

IF YOU KNOW WHERE TO LOOK!

Get the latest information on:
- **better health • diet & weight loss**
- **the latest nutritional supplements**
- **herbal healing • homeopathy and more**

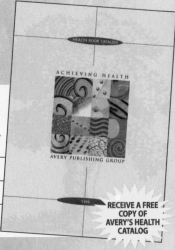

COMPLETE AND RETURN THIS CARD RIGHT AWAY!

Where did you purchase this book?

❑ bookstore ❑ health food store ❑ pharmacy
❑ supermarket ❑ other (please specify)_____

Name_____

Street Address_____

City_____State_____Zip_____

RECEIVE A FREE COPY OF AVERY'S HEALTH CATALOG

GIVE ONE TO A FRIEND ...

Healthy Habits

are easy to come by—

IF YOU KNOW WHERE TO LOOK!

Get the latest information on:
- **better health • diet & weight loss**
- **the latest nutritional supplements**
- **herbal healing • homeopathy and more**

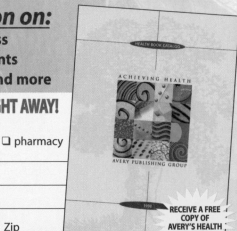

COMPLETE AND RETURN THIS CARD RIGHT AWAY!

Where did you purchase this book?

❑ bookstore ❑ health food store ❑ pharmacy
❑ supermarket ❑ other (please specify)_____

Name_____

Street Address_____

City_____State_____Zip_____

RECEIVE A FREE COPY OF AVERY'S HEALTH CATALOG

Avery Publishing Group
120 Old Broadway
Garden City Park, NY 11040

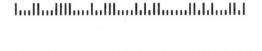

Avery Publishing Group
120 Old Broadway
Garden City Park, NY 11040